T0064470

Cosmic Energy and the Nature's Way in Health and Medicine

Cosmic Energy and the Nature's Way in Health and Medicine

KO PAANDU

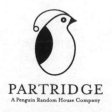

PARTRIDGE
A Penguin Random House Company

Copyright © 2015 by Ko Paandu.

ISBN: Hardcover   978-1-4828-5772-6
             Softcover   978-1-4828-5773-3
             eBook   978-1-4828-5771-9

All rights reserved. No part of this book may be used or reproduced by any means, graphic, electronic, or mechanical, including photocopying, recording, taping or by any information storage retrieval system without the written permission of the author except in the case of brief quotations embodied in critical articles and reviews.

Because of the dynamic nature of the Internet, any web addresses or links contained in this book may have changed since publication and may no longer be valid. The views expressed in this work are solely those of the author and do not necessarily reflect the views of the publisher, and the publisher hereby disclaims any responsibility for them.

Print information available on the last page.

To order additional copies of this book, contact
Partridge India
000 800 10062 62
orders.india@partridgepublishing.com

www.partridgepublishing.com/india

Contents

Acknowledgement vii

Preface ix

Introduction...xi

1. Life around 1

2. Around us 15

3. Cosmic Energy..31

4. Posions and Negions 42

5. Cosmic Energy in Health..59

6. Health and Disease 79

7. Food..103

8. Medicines..128

9. Herbs and Minerals...146

10. Chemicals 156

11. Energy in Medicine... 167

12. Energized medicine 181

13. Energy Activated to cure 195

14. Energy as Medicine.. 205

15. Old and New 211

16. Future 223

References 239

Acknowledgement

My grateful thanks go to my friend Dr. Pratul Kumar Chatterjea, environmental protection engineer, who introduced me to this subject on the influence of negative ions on human beings, when he offered me the books "Ion effect" by Fred Soyka and "Ion controversy" by Charles Wallah. These two books served as a beacon of light in directing my quest into uncharted areas while I have been seeking answers to several questions arising in my mind over the years.

I wish to record here my thanks to Mr. S.Sambamurthy, who has been of great assistance in reviewing this book from the start of this project till its submission as manuscript. His discussions, suggestions and analysis of certain critical subjects in the book helped me a great deal in realising the publication of this book.

I owe my thanks to my daughter Ms. P.Thenral, for her creative ideas in organising the subjects in the book and in its lucid presentation with illustrations. Timely reviews on the write-up and several new ideas suggested by my friend Mr. Ma.Elangovan were very helpful. I should thank my friends Mr. VR. Anbazhagan, Mr. S.Arul, Mr. L.Viswanathan, Mr. G.Gokulan, Mr. P.Senthil Murugan, Mr. V.Adithya and Mr. P.Venkatesan for their assistance in reviewing the manuscript. I owe my appreciation to Mr. M.Rajan for his detailed and thorough review of the manuscript and his valuable inputs.

The first to contact me from Partridge India was Mr. Maveric Pana after I showed my interest to get my book published. During that time the book was still in the conceptual level. A phone call from Ms. Racel Cruz served as a positive encouragement for me to exert myself more seriously from the slackened pace of writing at that time and commit myself with all seriousness to complete the project. I should thank Mr. Joe Anderson, who is the Associate with Partridge India for his close follow up to speed up my submissions for the publication.

Preface

Purpose of this book is to spread the awareness that nature has power, energy and remedy for all the living things on earth. Man need not create anything new once he learns how to use what is available in nature and respects and conserves nature for the future generations to come.

My friend, who is an Environmental Protection Engineer and Safety analyst by profession, gave me a book one day on our way to our office. When I started reading the book it appeared as if it was mirroring my own experiences here in India when compared with those of the author Fred Soyka in Geneva. The reality of events had a striking similarity and many of the experiences were similar during a natural phenomenon in Geneva as compared to my place in India. I could relate many conditions with certain type of environment at certain time period in Geneva and experienced similar environment during certain period of the year in South India. The book I got so deeply involved with is captioned as 'Ion effect' by Fred Soyka.

I was trying the allopathic medicine for my own health problem, which could not be resolved and was continuing for one year. In an unexpected circumstance I met an engineer, who used to prescribe alternative medicines for many health problems, as he pursued this activity as a hobby. The amount of medicine I had consumed was a little more than the size of a mustard seed and smaller than a pea and that too just one globule once a week. Improvement happened within a week and it created an interest in me to know what does it contain, how does it work, and in what way it is better than other medicines which could not solve my problems over one year. My knowledge in the field of medicine was quite poor and my interest on that subject faded in the years once my health problem had subsided.

When I read the book 'Ion effect', the uses of the natural energy re-kindled an interest in me to have some understanding on that wonder medicine that I chewed 10 years back. Then I realised that energy in material is the medicine and one need not know much about the medical world to understand and use the energized medicine to get the disease cleared from the body. Later I could understand by surfing the internet that energy itself is directly used to heal. Even though this system of medicine is not popular, it is spreading slowly among people, who now realise that there is a cure in that system of treatment.

The negative ions around us engulfed me and urged me to read whatever I could lay my hands on that subject and the result is this book on cosmic energy.

Introduction

'Cosmic Energy and the nature's way in Health and Medicine' is a book that explains the natural energy around us in everyday life and how we can maximize its use for our health. It also talks about how our health is connected with the body and mind and explains how disease is due to the disagreement between them.

This book explains the allergies and compares it with an enemy. One cannot solve a problem by avoiding the enemy. Largely an enemy would have been once a close friend. Same way allergy is the one you need to resolve and not avoid. Foodstuffs that were in use for centuries are what we are eating now and are the reliable to consume. Same way only the medicines that work consistently for at least a century could be reliable. The existing medicines do not endure even for a decade. There are many medicines proven for centuries and could help us to clear our diseases. This book brings out reasons as to why chemical medicines, herbs and minerals are not true medicines.

A medicine should act as an energized bullet or a piercing arrow which acts on the body and leaves the body. Instead chemical medicine stays in the body and becomes part of it creating hell of a lot of side effects. A medicine is supposed to cure the disease of the person and not create a disease basket accumulating more diseases. On the other hand only the energized medicines which are slow but steady can clear our disease at nature's speed and not the fast acting palliative medicines.

1

Life around

Our fast life and activity
makes us
think that the life of
everybody and everything
around us is also fast.
We do not have time to look around

When life was slow
we thought outside is also slow.
We did our work slowly
and
found time
to watch around us
and
lived in harmony with nature

Life in a day of Kumaar:

His father was admitted in the hospital for about a week and was in the Intensive Care Unit. The doctor told Kumaar that his father did not need any more hospitalisation and could move back to his house. Kumaar's father was asthmatic and was having breathing problem. The old man was on oxygen support for some time. Doctor told Kumaar that his father would be fine if he starts breathing fresh air. Doctor advised Kumaar to ensure that the room where his father would stay should be made dust free and explained that the old man's suffering may be due to dust allergy.

What way fresh air and that too the air very much contaminated by pollution is going to improve the health and not the pure and clean oxygen of the hospital?

Kumaar brought his father home with a healthier improvement in his condition. The old man was visibly happy and enthusiastic to be back in his room and with his grand children. Soon, another subject needed Kumaar's urgent attention after his father's health. Kumaar, who is fifty years old, has a son and daughter. The son, who

> **Month named 'Aaadi'** in Tamil calendar used in South Indianstate of Tamilnadu (pronounced as Tamilnaadu). Day one of the month Aadi is around July15th in Gregarian Calendar

is older of the two is married and has two kids aged, eight and four. The daughter is working as a teacher at a local school, after a degree in education training. It was time for Kumaar to seek a marriage alliance for his daughter and the subject was getting postponed due to the ailment of his father. The old man used to say 'I will die only after witnessing the marriage of my granddaughter. Kumaar wanted to arrange the marriage as early as possible and was on the lookout for a suitable groom.

Kumaar was advised by his uncle about a possible alliance for his daughter in a town about forty kilometres away. Kumaar called up the family of the bridegroom and set up the meeting. The family is related to him through his mother's side and he finds no problem to set up his meeting. However he has to hurry up to reach a decision within two days before the advent of the Tamil calendar month, 'Aadi'.

In what way the month called 'Aadi' of Tamil calendar has anything to do with his daughter's marriage or to initiate talks with her future in-law's family?

Kumaar works as an administrative manager in a textile firm. He had taken leave from his office for five days due to the hospitalisation of his father. Kumaar planned for a bus travel next day and slept with the thought of his father and about his important activities from dawn to dusk the following day. He planned to travel early morning and return by evening since he should attend his office on the following day.

> **Arranged marriages** are common in India, the discussions on those subjects will take place during 'good time' and 'good day' based on Panchaangam, a book of astronomy calculations.
>
> In Tamilnadu, an astrology book is used as reference for fixing auspicious dates and times for social and family events. Not everybody believes in this practice but it has become a custom followed by many over the years.

Next day he got up early and took leave of his wife and went to the bus terminal and boarded the bus. All his thoughts in the bus were about his family and mainly the marriage. His Office issues were less demanding as he had the requisite skills in administration. His son had been working as an engineer for a construction company and his job was a routine supervision in recent months. In the absence of Kumaar, his son used to take care of his grandfather.

The travel, by direct bus from Kumaar's town to the town of the perspective bridegroom was not so tiresome. He met the parents of future bridegroom and discussions went on smoothly. Bridegroom's father wanted a copy of bride's horoscope and Kumaar had already carried one with him in anticipation. Kumaar had the horoscope of the prospective groom in advance. He had already ascertained from the astrologer about the compatibility of the bride and groom and only then decided to start discussions with the groom's family.

The two parties decided to have further talks after the month of *'Aadi'*. Kumaar was told by the groom's parents that they would be able to see their astrologer the next day and would convey the outcome as soon as possible. Only on confirmation from groom's family after the family astrologer's go ahead, Kumaar would be in a position to make arrangements to fix the date and venue for the wedding. However, even after the possible confirmation for the alliance, Kumaar would need to wait for a whole month (*Aadi*) to pass before he could proceed with preparations for the marriage.

On his way back Kumaar decided to visit a temple to offer his prayers to God to bless his daughter with a positive result from the groom's side astrologer and for a happy married life. The temple is situated on the top of a small hill. One has to climb on foot around three hundred steps to reach the top of the hill. Kumaar could climb the steps, even though he was a bit slow. The temple is a small one and it did not take him much time to go around the temple and complete his prayers.

Temple visits

It is customary to visit temples and offer prayers prior to any important occasions in the family.

Why many temples, churches and even houses, which are built on hill tops has attraction for the people in spite of the efforts to climb the steps. Is the attraction more towards structures on the hill or mountain compared to those at the ground level?

He felt peace and comfort after the visit to the temple. He could not think of any reason for his positive feelings. Whenever any event is planned at his household, Kumaar usually used to visit this temple to offer prayers. He descended down the steps of the hill and had his lunch at a restaurant. He had politely refused food in the house of his future groom as it is a customary practice not to have food at the home of prospective in-laws before a marriage is finalised. Kumaar had instead replied with optimism to his relative that he will enjoy the meals later on when marriage is settled.

The trip from the town of the temple back to his home town was again by bus travel. He got into the bus and was soon immersed in his thoughts once again on the events of that day, as the bus started moving and the noises of the bus terminal faded away. This particular route does not have any train link. Hence he had to travel both ways by bus and fortunately bus connections

Bus Travel vs Train Travel:

Travel comfort has the difference when travel by car, bus, truck or Train. Trains have metal contact with the earth whereas other road transport vehicles have tires, which is not electrically conductive. This makes the difference in the uneasiness by bus travel.

were convenient with good frequency of service. Kumaar felt more comfortable whenever he travelled by train and his travel to the big cities were usually by train. However during his bus journey he used to feel uneasy and would wait for the halts en route where bus usually stops for five to ten minutes. He used to get down from the bus and take a stroll for a while and then get in. So was the practice with some other passengers too. On the other hand, he found train travel as comfortable and never felt the need to get out till he reaches his destination. In case a bus stops at a restaurant for food, invariably everybody gets out and gets in even if they do not consume any food in the restaurants. This time the bus did not stop in any restaurant.

Many passengers feel uncomfortable when travelling by bus. Why? Journey by train never gives passengers that kind of stress. Why?

It is by now around 2 p.m. and the climate was quite hot and humid. He expected that it might rain within next couple of hours. Suddenly the onset of thunder and lightning that lit the skies shook him out of his thoughts. It was earlier than he had anticipated. The heat and humidity had gone and a tense situation was felt during lightning and thunder. He always felt tensed up before travel and that too when lightning and thunder were close by. His wife and son used to poke fun at him when they noticed such feeling in him. To avoid the embarrassment Kumaar started to breathe deeply not to show his tension. He has an underlying fear for the thunder that he could not overcome.

The rain started as a slow drizzle at first and the drops increased, but the rain was not heavy. The bus reached Kumaar's town but still the rain continued. Kumaar disembarked from the bus and waited under the shade of the bus stop shelter. Rain continued and the rain drops brought a cool feeling and he was enjoying an air-conditioned atmosphere, while his mind was with thoughts of that day, by now each thought linking with future extension. The rain brought the smell of the soil from the nearby fields around the town.

Why do some people tense up during lightning or thunder but feel subsequently relaxed during the rain?

Soon Kumaar reached his home and the rain had stopped by now. He decided to clean up the room for his father as he had no time to attend to this before he left his home, the priority being the marriage of his daughter. Kumaar started removing the surplus goods that was gathering dust for months in his father's room. He could realise that the dust would have caused more harm and breathing difficulties to his ailing father.

How come just dust and pollen can cause or accentuate Asthmatic symptoms?

Do all the following subjects which are not necessarily related to one another in the above events have something in common?

- Fresh air instead of oxygen for a patient
- An inauspicious month to avoid auspicious discussions
- A temple on a hill top attracts more pilgrims
- Train travel is more comfortable than bus.
- Thunder and lightning creating stress in some people
- Rain showers promote relaxation of the mind
- Dust allergy aggravates asthma
- Dust affects a few people selectively

You may be surprised that all the above apparently unconnected subjects have something in common to connect. Many of us experience them but never got a feeling that there could be a link, still even if thinking arises we find no time to analyse or have no capability to correlate. Many of the events above are experienced by many- You, me and even our neighbour in day to day life.

Some events experienced by our forefathers over a long period of times caused them to devise certain customs for their future generation to follow. Some customs remain in force and are still being followed, although many of us do not know the reasons of those customs. Some customs and practices are modified by succeeding generations and others followed blindly without any meaning or use. Some of the customs advised by our forefathers may be in good interest, learnt out of their experience and may be with good outcomes. We do not follow them as we do not reason out the meaning behind those customs.

Even science might not have related the events that we and our forefathers are experiencing and have experienced. Present science may not have the answers now, but future will not stay same. The above events of nature that create the thoughts, feeling and effects on humans are not in the realm of science at the moment. It is said that they have not been 'scientifically proven'. However some scientists have started giving reasons for the above events and are helping others to utilise their benefits.

What is science? Observation, Formation of a Hypothesis, Theory or a Rule is the sequence in science. All observations on that specific category would agree with the formulated hypothesis. The formulae and equations fit perfectly in physics and chemistry due to the research of scientists. By experience, the minute errors were cleared and perfections brought by time. That is science, which is composed of measurements, readings and records.

Many such observations by human, animal and plant senses may not be able to be measured and matched to some hypothesis. Human observation is built into experience and it shaped the life of the society. Slowly the society started living based on the experience of others. Individuals started following the society and education and science reduced the need for observations and formulating theories. This resulted in meagre inventions in the basics of life, nature and environment. Most of the new researches by the scientists are over and above the existing concepts and repetitions. The new thinking even with new observations has become very limited. The reason is the thinking itself is channelized by education by teaching 'How to think'. The free thinking is reducing and basic theories are in saturation even though there could be lot in nature to be brought into science.

When a child is born and separated from the mother immediately after birth, the mother cannot always identify her baby. But a sheep can identify the calf even in the crowd of sheep by some sense of smell. The reason may be that we lost the sense of smell but the animals did not. Animals are with nature and the nature makes them learn to survive.

When will science investigate and form hypothesis and theories for events like Silva Method of mind training, one of the most powerful systems of self help techniques. Out-of-body and near-death experiences are presented by Edgar Cayce, known as "The Sleeping Prophet", "America's Greatest Mystic" and palmistry by the most famous hand reader in history, Cheiro are yet to come under a theory. Water diviners could locate the water streams down below the earth. The phenomenon above may be termed as paranormal or parapsychology but should be equated to the principle of science. Human observation and thinking has to go deeper and deeper to find the equations and solutions and there may be a limit also for these micro or nano observations.

The human race has lost many senses through the course of channelized education. Science need not prove everything and cannot prove it either. Science has limitations based on its equipments, measuring capabilities, etc. Experiences of animals and plants may extend beyond the limit of human observations, more in the area where science cannot measure. Furthermore happens in the area where humans cannot observe but animals can sense. Beyond animals there could be more and more signals where even plants can sense (Tompkins, 2002).

The police use dogs to sniff out the drugs and also to trace the paths of robbers. Animals sense the rain, earthquakes and any natural events easily and scientists are yet to device the theories and formulae to explain these.

People who have no access to the science may be still in the Stone Age but live with nature and have their old basic sense retained with them. Years back during the tsunami of Indonesia on 24th December 2004, natives of the Andaman Islands in the Bay of Bengal Sea could escape to top of mountains and the non-natives perished in the towns.

Many scientists have proved some of the facts, beyond the present science, but cannot propagate their findings to the people. The reason being Science Psychology, called science addiction. Once any scientific information, embedded in our consciousness, the perception never changes easily and we feel that as our final understanding and that is the right one to follow. Another idea in science is to enter into our consciousness and change the concept to the core. Science does this tortuous task and the success depends on the individuals' acceptance or rejection. Our human race is inculcated to follow the society. We believe the science of that time when we are told or we read that this is 'scientifically proved' and 'science has established the facts'. When an advertisement is broadcasted that 98% of people get well by medicine xyz, et cetera we start consuming it. Why? What is the reason to believe in science blindly? It is an educational addiction. After few years same science would tell us that the medicine xyz produces lot of side effects leading to bad health conditions. Only then, the government starts announcing its plan to ban the medicine even then the same governments never care to implement these actions.

Think of Penicillin as an example. Penicillin is one of the first and also one of the most widely used antibiotic. Discovered by bacteriologist Alexander Fleming in 1928 this was the best antibiotic and saved many lives and mainly of soldiers during the Second World War. Penicillin came to medicine industry in mass scale only in 1943 and started its side effects by 1947 within 20 years of its invention. Microbes started resisting the drug producing toxins in the body and side effects like pneumonia. In 2005 US FDA (Food and Drug Administration) banned the penicillin in poultry industry.

How do we differentiate different theories of science for the same subject with a gap of few years? That is the experience of science. Any invention is popularised the instant it gets attraction and we believe it and follow it. For example they promoted the synthetic fertilisers are best and food production would make the world poverty zero. Few years passed. Same scientists propagate now not to use synthetic fertilisers and advice us to go for organic agriculture with natural manure. What was researched by few scientists years back have to be proved wrong by the experience of many. Now the theory we have learned had to be unlearned. Again after few years the concepts on same subject may change and we may have to unlearn and learn. How to differentiate the two theories? Which is wrong? The old or the new? How come one medicine that was good a few years back is bad now? Now we have to learn that what was good is now no good. May be after some years this medicine may be considered good. We accept the latest as correct, not learning but following.

Our life continued for centuries without any science. Life improved only by experience and that experience recorded by a few as observations and then theories in science. It helped us to learn more and more and that started binding us making us forget our own experience. Also the same science has slowly started to watch the entry of anything new in science to be rejected or opposed if hinders the existing business or cultural or individual interests. Even the proven experiments on biological transmutations by scientists like Kervran and others were rejected by other science groups (Jean-Paul-2012). The science has been taken over by business.

Science may not have the instruments and tools to measure many observations. The incapability to measure would ignore the observations as non-science or parascience. There is tremendous scope for science to learn from nature and the area of research is wide open; when one is able to measure the very low frequency of thoughts and very high frequencies of electromagnetic spectrum, when one is able to measure the very low light intensity near to dark and high intensity of lightning, when one is able to measure very low currents of our body and high currents of lightning and when one can measure the distance between the particles in atom and distances between objects in space. The limit for measurement has no limit and one day science may be able to record the observations if science community helps the society to that level of knowledge and intelligence.

When is the science going to find theories for so many observations prevailing around us? How long and how deep the science could be going into the thinking, assessing, analysing, judging and deciding on the events in the life of day to day human activity. The life now is beyond the grip of science for understanding. The grip of science is mathematics, a human invention. Next is physics and chemistry connected with materials using the calculations in mathematics. With all the great developments in science how come engineering theories hold good for years and medical sciences are changing day by day and even today inventing medicines behind diseases.

We do not know how long the science could take to bring the Biological sciences to its control.

Practices in human society instead of bringing people closer to each other to live in love and harmony have started dividing them. Then again reunite them in the name of mother's day, father's day and even to remember and recall a lover on a valentine's day. These special days are devised as a means to substitute genuine thoughts and emotions which have been lost in time from natural day to day activities in our social fabric. This is the way we spoil first and then rectify in all spheres of human life.

Police and home security systems are there to install cameras which serve as deterrents or to help capture the face of thieves in order to help in arresting them. Years back the same police advocated to use a hard door, strong gate so that robbers do not enter. Many years back people were cultured enough to be good in society not to want others wealth.

Like fences for a land, rules are made for a society. More rules cause the society not to think but to follow something blindly. This is nothing but sheep following other sheep. As already mentioned people are coached on how to think nowadays. It means the basic thinking process is in the path of decay.

We talk about health more after losing it. 'Prevention is better than cure' if practiced widely cannot earn money for the medical business. Hence taking medicine is promoted as the better way now to ensure good health than taking good food. Eating sweets and taking a diabetic pill is the norm of life of the day.

Let us go back to the day of Kumaar's. What is that which is common in a day's events for Kumaar and has that much impact on all living things that is part of atmospheric air?

They are negative ions, negatively charged particles and have a charge equivalent to electrons. These negative ions are called also as Negions or NAI (Negative Air Ions).

Oxygen gives energy to the body by energizing the cells. Negative ions feed energy to the mind. The energy that is the base for our life is just around without us knowing it. The energy is around us and engulfing us.

There is a force in the universe,
which, if we permit it,
will flow through us and
produce miraculous results

-Mahatma Gandhi-

2

Around us

Our life goes on.
Everything around us goes on
whether we are active or not

We may know what is around us.
But we do not know
why they are like that
and what they can do
the reason is
the fast paced life

Nature
in a few moments
changes the
surrounding environment
around us
very fast
without us being aware of it.

Comfort for you and your body:

When you are sitting in a room you feel uncomfortable at times even when you are not sweating and with the right temperature and humidity. If the size of the room is small you are more likely to feel uneasiness and discomfort. The feeling arises less often if the room is large and with a high roof. You may feel that the room is air-conditioned flawlessly and adequate amount of air is available to breathe but why should you still feel stuffy?

What happens in reality?

Even when the same temperature and humidity prevails in different rooms with the same cleanliness you may not feel the same level of comfort in all the rooms. Sometimes we say fresh air circulation is missing. If the room is maintained to be clean and with fresh air circulated with the air-conditioning system with an optimal temperature and humidity no uneasy feeling is supposed to come up. At the same time when you stand outside the room and in the open atmosphere with same climatic conditions your feeling is awesome. Why?

The Simple reason is that the feeling of wellbeing is dependent on outside air, which has something to do within you in energizing you to make you comfortable in feeling and physical presence. Room air conditioners and HVAC systems are designed to allow a small quantity of outside air. Some HVAC (Heating, Ventilation and Air-Conditioning) systems are not designed to add sufficient outside air to the re-circulated ventilation system. Why do you need outside air circulation when the surrounding air has the correct temperature with the required air flow around your body and the air is humid within comfortable limits? Think for a while. There is something which we are not aware but it makes us feel comfortable when outside air is mixed with the re-circulated air. The re-circulated air had some energized particles at the start which gets consumed by the people in the rooms. The charged particles in the air were creating the comfort and clearing the uneasy feeling in us.

The experience is more dramatic when a crowd gathers in an auditorium. There is freshness when few people arrive and gather in the hall. Being a big hall or theatre the atmosphere is good. People start gathering. The event starts in time, the program continues and slowly people feel the suffocation. At first nobody feels the itch. The clock ticks and everybody starts consuming the energy in the atmosphere from air present and the refilling of fresh air is limited. Our assumption is the oxygen consumption from our knowledge of science. We are not aware of the reduction of negative ions, the cosmic energy. We think oxygen is consumed. This does not happen where there is less of a crowd or a good amount of circulation of outside air mixed with conditioned air (Wallach, 2010).

The charged particles in the atmospheric air create the comfort what the temperature and humidity cannot produce the same in you. The charged particles that create the comfort are called NEGATIVE IONS. The atmospheric air also contains POSITIVE IONS. The imbalance between the charges creates the discomfort. The balance is when positive ions and negative ions are within a specific proportions. The imbalance is caused when positive ions are increased in ratio to the negative ions.

The extra entity in the air, that promotes the good feeling are the negative ions. You start consuming the negions (Negative ions) in the air and needs re-filling. The re-circulated air in the room never brings the same quality as fresh air which contains the negative ions. Better than the re-circulated air in the room, a step into the outside environment brings more comfort because of the availability of negative ions.

All the suffocation is due to insufficient negions in the closed room.

When a person gets up early in the morning, there is freshness at sunrise and the same person when he gets up after a nap in the evening, he feels dull. One can notice this when his or her house is built with its front facing east the morning, causing them to be cheerful. Many temples are built facing towards the east. Many prayers are performed by looking at the morning sun.

Any time of an event, when the event faces many obstacles while it is conducted or the end objective is not achieved is considered as bad time or inauspicious. Some people believe in good and bad times in a day. Then what is the good time or auspicious time and how do we determine one? The good and bad times are learnt by gaining experience over a long period covered by several generations. Experience of a person with nature is not his age or years he dwelt in that place or locality but the years the person's forefathers and his generation learned over the years in that geographical area with the surrounding atmosphere, vegetation, people, natural events etc.

The same atmosphere which gives energy also creates problems too to the health. There are many dry winds or 'Witches' winds in different parts of the world. In nature, at many places on earth, the air, though may not be contaminated or polluted, develops an imbalance due to the electrical charges of the particles in the air. The dry wind may be hot or cold but charges of the ionic particles in the air changes. It happens mainly in places where the air flow is channelled by mountains and air rifts with the sides of the mountain and the valley. These winds are typically warm and dry. The air currents occur where mountains stand in the path of strong air flow. The rubbing of air along the slopes of the mountains creates the electrical charges in the particles in air. This is like rubbing the palms of one's hand that produces lift of hair due to build up of static charges. One such major wind is from the European Alps and is known as the Foehn, a poison wind. A similar wind occurs in India too called Aadi wind during the Tamil calendar month of Aaadi. This has been explained in the previous chapter and how it plays a little part in the life of Kumaar.

Why the winds are named? Any important subject is named as it plays a major role in the part of human life. The wind which are normal and that does not affect us much goes unnoticed without anybody's curiosity. The winds get a name when they are famous or notorious in causing discomfort, havocs, disasters and problems to the community. More attention is given to any factor when it causes a problem that affects us deep within.

Like the **Aadi** wind in Southern India during July-August many *Witches'* winds exist throughout the world as compiled and briefed below.

Bise wind in Geneva, Switzerland is a cold, vigorous and persistent north or north-easterly wind blowing from the alpine mountains. This affects Switzerland and eastern France. The city of Geneva, sits on narrow V-shaped plain between Lake Geneva and the point where Alps converge. The Bise is especially prominent in the Geneva area at the south western end of Lake Geneva. Fred Soyka describes his health experience in Geneva due to such dry atmosphere in his book 'Ion effect'. The Bise whips up the surface waters of Lake Geneva and in winter the sea spray encases the nearby vegetation under thick ice. During summer the dry Bise is a perfect laundry drier finding its reflection in the local folklore: "avec la bise, lave ta chemise", when the Bise blows, wash your shirt. During the dry season when winds create uneasy atmosphere and discomfort, people move to the rural areas. Doctors too are busy in this season due to bad health condition of inhabitants.

Foehn **in Geneva, Switzerland,** is different from Bise and this dehydrated, warm and dry wind is from southeast touching the surface of the mountains and hitting the valley, the lake and the city. *Foehn* is a condition rather than the state. The state is felt only after the positively charged particles are left in the city in packets. These charges create a build up of static electricity and stays for long even after the wind dies down. In the 19th century, Austrian physician, Anton Czermak published a clinical review of the effects of Foehn as the residents in areas of frequent Foehn winds were reporting illnesses ranging from migraines to psychosis. Also a study by the University of Munich (Ludwig-Maximilians-Universität-München) found that suicide and accidents increased by 10 percent during Foehn winds in Central Europe.

Foehn in Munich, Germany and Austria, is a generic term for warm, strong and often very dry down slope winds that descend in the lee side of a mountain barrier. *Foehn* (föhn in German) type winds are known for their rapid temperature rise, their desiccating effect and the rapid disappearance of snow cover. Due to the similarity in condition that prevails over the land and people after the wind, other such winds in different parts of the world are called ***Foehn*** winds.

Tramontane in France is a strong, dry cold wind from the north or from the northwest. And on the Mediterranean, the *tramontane* is created by the difference of pressure between the cold air of a high pressure system over the northwest Europe and a low pressure over the Gulf of Lion in the Mediterranean. The high-pressure air flows south, gathering speed as it moves. The continuous howling noise of the *tramontane* is said to have a disturbing effect upon the human psyche. Victor Hugo, in his poem, the main character says "The wind coming over the mountain will drive me mad..."

The **Mistral** in France is a strong, cold and north westerly wind that blows from southern France into the Gulf of Lion in the northern Mediterranean. The mistral (meaning 'mud eater'), though it blows in all seasons, occurs mainly in winter or spring. It lasts only one or two days and sometimes continues for days more than a week. It has a major influence all along the Mediterranean coast of France and frequently causes sudden storms in the Mediterranean. The **mistral** is usually accompanied by clear and fresh weather, which plays an important role in creating the climate of the region and bringing good health. The dry air dries stagnant water and the mud and blows away the pollution from the skies over the large cities and industrial areas. The mistral also saves crops from the spring frost. Also the sunshine and dryness carried by the mistral wind has an important effect on the local vegetation. The vegetation which is already due to shortage of rainfall is made even drier. By this, vegetation is more prone to fire and once fire starts the wind escalates the fire. The mistral causes irritating headaches and mothers complain the wind provokes restlessness in children. Some pet keepers complain that pets are affected by this wind.

Bora in the Adriatic is a northern to north-eastern wind in Montenegro, Italy, Bulgaria, Greece, Slovenia, Bosnia, Croatia, Herzegovina, Bulgaria, Greece, Poland and southwest part of Russia. In Croatian the wind is called "burno", which means "violently" and is commonly used to describe the weather. Bora is a cold and very dry wind. These winds occur any time in a year but mostly in the cold season and lasts from few days to a month.

Halny wind in Poland blows in south Poland and in Slovakia in the Carpathian Mountains. Wind comes from South on one side, down the slopes of the Tatra Mountains; in Slovakia and from North, the other side of the mountains. Most *Halny* occur in October and November, sometimes in February and March, rarely in other months. *Halny* is a warm wind through the valleys and often is a disastrous one. It causes avalanches, lifts the roofs of homes and according to some people, can have some influence on the mental state of some people like the ***Foehn*** wind.

Sirocco in North Africa is the name for the hot and humid wind in some parts of North Africa and has many names in each region. Along the northern African coast the hot air originates directly from the Sahara desert, producing hot, dry and dusty conditions. The desert-air over Northern Africa, flows northward into the southern Mediterranean basin. Visibility becomes very poor and the fine blowing dust might result in damage permeating into the instruments and equipments. On rare occasions the Sirocco is picking up enough dust and sand to produce even sandstorms. Sirocco creates a cool wet weather in Europe. The wind is mainly in March and November and touches a speed of 100 km/h (Kilometres per hour) at its peak. Sirocco creates a depressive feeling among people during the wind season.

The Sirocco has different characteristics and has many different local names, too. The term Sirocco is not used in North Africa, where it is called **chom** (hot) or **arifi** (thirsty); **Simoom** in Palestine, Jordan, Syria, and the desert of Arabia; **Ghibli** or **leveche** (or Chibli, Gibla, Gibleh) in Libya; **Chili** (or Chichili) in Tunisia and Algeria; **Sharav** in Israel; **Ikslok** in Mediterranean; **Khamsin** (or Chamsin, Khamasseen) in Egypt and around the Red Sea.

The Old Testament calls the Middle Eastern *Sharav* an evil, destructive and deceiving wind in one of its translations.

Sirocco in Europe affects the southern Mediterranean basin. It has the same demoralised feeling that prevails in North African region. The bad health conditions of individuals create troubles between people.

Simoon in Sahara and Arabian Desert is a very hot, dry, suffocating wind combined with dust that swings across the African deserts, mainly Arabia, Syria, Jordan and its neighbouring countries. *Simoon* creates extreme heat in the prevailing arid deserts and the sandy plains. *Simoon* lasts less than half an hour and brings up the dust and sand from the floor of the desert. *Simoon* is not the main wind. This a secondary wind with the result of thermal heating of the dry surface. This wind reshapes the terrain and forms sand dunes too. The name comes from the Arabic '*samma*' for Poison. It is also called *Samiel* in some regions.

Khamsin (fifty) in North Africa is a Fifty day wind is an oppressive, hot, dry and dusty south or south-east wind occurring in North Africa, around the East Mediterranean and the Arabian Peninsula intermittently in late winter and early summer, but most frequently between April and June. A counterpart of the sirocco, it is a southerly wind over Egypt blowing from the Sahara Desert and an easterly over the Negev Desert and parts of Saudi Arabia. The term is also applied to very strong southerly or south-westerly winds over the Red Sea. Less frequently the *khamsin* might also occur in winter as a cold, dusty wind.

Santa Ana winds in California is the seasonal strong wind in Southern California, which is hot, dry and dusty. The Santa Ana winds originate from inland sweeping down from the deserts and across coastal southern California, pushing dust and smoke of forest fires far out to the Pacific Ocean. Santa Ana winds blow mostly in autumn and winter, but can arise at other times of the year also. They can range from hot to cold, depending on the prevailing temperatures in the source regions. The winds are known especially for the hot dry weather, often the hottest of the year and are infamous for fanning regional wildfires. For these reasons, they are sometimes known as the "devil winds" across Southern California.

It is widely believed in Southern California that the winds affect people's moods and behavior negatively. Even without ironclad scientific proof, it is a well-accepted part of local lore. There is some belief the winds also create positive ions, which are believed to affect mood negatively. Many believe this to be the cause for the statistical increase in the number of suicides and homicides during these times. The Santa Ana wind becomes a part of novels too like the "Red wind" by Raymond Chandler and Ross MacDonald. American Indians, according to their mythology, call the Santa Ana wind as Bitter Winds. The folklore tells of people's wind sickness when they get exposed to the Bitter Winds.

Chinooks in US blow across much of the North American states, particularly the Rocky Mountain region during the winter months. Statistical studies point out that during these winds, road accidents happen more frequently and suicide rates increase. Hospitals postpone some operations and wait for the winds to calm down.

Chinook in Canada, interior West of North America refers to the winds where Canadian Prairies and Great Plains meet various mountain ranges. The name Chinook for the wind is derived from the name of the people of that region, along the lower Columbia River. A strong Chinook can make snow one foot deep almost vanish in one day. Chinook winds have been observed to raise winter temperature, often from below -20 °C (-4 °F) to as high as 10-20 °C (50-68 °F). This used to last for a few hours or few days and then the temperatures plunges to their base levels. Chinook winds, sometimes, are said to cause a sharp increase in the number of migraine headaches suffered by the locals, and are often called "chinook headaches". At least one study conducted by the department of clinical neurosciences at the University of Calgary supports that belief. They are popularly believed to increase irritability and sleeplessness. Many migraine sufferers believe changes in weather can trigger migraines.

Thar desert, Rajasthan-India, has hot and dry environment is due to the isolation of desert by the mountain ranges and plains. This contributes significantly to the weather patterns that shape its distinctive environment around the desert. The desert effectively absorbs all the moisture that is carried in the monsoon clouds before the clouds can reach the desert. The resulting monsoon winds in the desert are hot and dry. Wind activity over Thar Desert is at low ebb during the winters. From March onwards when the surface is dry and temperatures soar the summer winds associated with south west monsoon reach a maximum speed of 20 km per hour or more. Advancing summers further dry up the ground and whatever vegetation tried to grow in the winters is dry by May. The arrival of monsoon in July puts an end to this activity.

Aadi Kaatru (*Aadi* wind) in South India is popular due to the dry atmosphere it creates with dullness among people. The wind force is high and there is a proverb in that region which says "The wind of Aadi can even move a grinding stone used in kitchen". The wind used to be with shrill noise. This is the season for the Southwest monsoon. In case the rain joins the wind the damages would be high. The monsoon has two branches of winds Arabian Sea Branch and the Bay of Bengal Branch near the southernmost end of the Indian Peninsula. The wind hails from Bay of Bengal travels on the eastern side of the mountains of Western Ghats. This is mostly a dry wind. The Arabian Sea branch carries the moisture of the sea and blows towards North creating a good rainy atmosphere in North India up to the foothills of Himalayas. The wind from the Arabia Sea travels west of the mountains in Kerala but drags the wind of Bay of Bengal. This wind dragged rubs along the mountain bordering Tamil Nadu. The wind blows in northern direction and travels a long stretch of the hills. The air carries heavy dust sometimes forces the people to stay indoors. The wind is forceful during July and August and sometimes with rains. Due to the dry wind bad mood prevails in most of the parts of South Indian Peninsula.

Aadi is considered the windiest month and so there is a greater chance of fire accidents. Industrial sources say most of the major fire accidents happened in Aadi. The farmers in southern part of India, after a monsoon rain and ploughing, do the sowing in mid-August, i.e. end of month called 'Aadi' in Tamil calendar. This sowing time is by experience and there is a proverb "Do the sowing waiting for the *Aadi* season". Why the sowing is exactly at this time is another question (Srikumar-2014)?

This atmospheric condition of month *Aadi* (mid July to mid August) is dry and is full of *Witches* winds throughout south India. No important event would take place during this month. Hence it is considered as an inauspicious month too. No major decisions on any event would be discussed in the family. During this period family functions, carnivals, temple functions, business deals or marriages will be avoided. Even decisions or discussions on events like marriages are avoided. Newly married couple would not be allowed to live together as husband and wife (Sankaran, 2014).

What is the reason for these?

The month called '*Aadi*' has dry winds with dust supplying the atmosphere of southern India with more positive ions than negative ions. This causes the mind to dull and hence a system is followed not to decide major life concerned decisions are either delayed or postponed. Any decision would be before or after this inauspicious month.

With all this negativity about Aadi, why the sowing is done in that month of Aadi? The sowing done at the end of the month of Aadi makes a better germination due to positive ions and sprouts protrude the soil smoothly. Positive ions have important effect over the germination of seeds and negative ions help in the plant growth. After this month of Aadi, the atmosphere changes with full of negative ions and helps to grow the plant.

Like Bise, Foehn, Tramontane, Bora, Sirocco, Simoon, Khamsin, Santa Ana winds, Chinook, Thar desert wind and Addi Kaatru these winds in different parts of the globe has the same but similar characteristic of the Foehn wind of Europe. These winds have other names in many other regions: Zonda in Argentina, Koembang in Java, Warm Braw in Schouten Islands off the north coast of New Guinea and Oroshi in Japan.

Health effects of the winds - Good and Bad:

You may wonder how different types of winds at different weather conditions affect our health and mainly the mental conditions. The warm, dry wind is likely to drain the energy of the people making them suffer in their daily life. *Witches* Winds have been blamed for making the people bad-tempered, irritable, prickly, depressed, tired, sleepy and unhappy. The same have also been blamed for increased quarrels, traffic accidents, murders and suicides. Many countries suffer due to the winds of their landscape. All the troubles are mind related and reflected in the body too. The winds themselves are problems to the damage of properties etc. and the effect on people's mental depression is due to the content of the wind, the high value of positive ions compared to the negative ions. It is the imbalance of ions, the molecules of air within the winds that are so frustrating and annoying.

These invisible ions are inhaled and also adsorbed through the skin. They are either positively or negatively charged. When the air has too many positive ions, which are 1,800 times heavier than negative ones, it becomes dry and heavy. The best balance is 5 positive ions to 4 negative ions. The ion discharge due to formation of clouds during lightning and also just before the storm formation increases the posions. An increase of positive ions compared to negative ions makes us moody, out of sorts and lethargic during those periods. We can feel the refreshing effect after the storm passes due to reduction of posions compared to negions. That's because the heavy positive ions were carried away by rain drops and cleaned away. At the same time of rain plenty of negative ions are generated. The negative ion increase is due to the interaction of rain drops with air. Best balanced ratio of Negion to Posion would be 0.8 and would be very much down to 0.3 before the storm and the negions would increase to 3 times that of posions after the storm and during rain (Wallah, 2010).

Many hill and mountain areas, seashores and waterfalls produce large amounts of negative ions. Yosemite Valley, California, has one of the most negative ion-filled environments in the state. In New York and Canada, Niagara Falls has been called the most immense negative ion generator in the world. In our homes, a great negative ion generator is the bath room shower.

What does the dry atmosphere creates in the health of the people of that region? The Swiss Meteorological Institute made an extensive study in 1974 and published the problems arising from *Foehn* type wind. Above all, these winds can make us seem bad and short-tempered, argumentative and quarrelsome without any clear reason. Also this makes us think that we are in good mood even though it is not so. The Table-1 lists the problems in various places.

Table-1. What Posions create and subsequent effects during witches' winds.

Winds causes	Subsequent effects
Anxiety and tension	Leading cause for bad decisions
Catching cold	No patience to wait and creates interest for medication
Lassitude, sleeplessness or bad sleep	Lethargy
Depression	Lethargy
Reduced sex drive	Broken marriages
Changing moods	Non cohesive decisions
One day optimistic next day depressed	Alternating moods
Exhaustion	Higher incidence of heart attacks
Respiratory problems	Asthma
Irritability	Slower reaction time
Body pains	Joint pains
Sick headaches	Nausea, stuffy nose
Variations in body salts - sodium, calcium and magnesium	Dizziness

When the dry winds die down they leave another effect due to the static electricity. Static electricity is formed due to accumulated concentration of charged particles at one place. Positive ions being a heavy particles and also has attraction

towards the negative earth. The accumulated charges create
an electric field. This is similar to a state of high voltage
system creating an electric field. These electric fields create
disturbances in biological systems.

A build-up of static electricity occurs due to the accumulation
negative ions or positive ions. Individuals can feel static
electricity when they touch the metallic door knob after a walk
over synthetic carpets. Bad ventilations in computer rooms
also create static charges and hence floor carpeting are done
for them with anti-static properties, carpets ingrained with
metallic fibres and connected to the floor.

To overcome all the bad effects of the atmosphere and *Witches*
winds, nature provides us with abundance of negative ions,
called **Cosmic Energy.**

My brain is only a receiver, in the universe there is a core
from which we obtain knowledge, strength and inspiration.
I have not penetrated into the secrets of
this core, but I know it exists.

-Nikola Tesla-

3

Cosmic Energy

Earth is just a dot
in this vast boundless universe.

Our life and life of everything
in the cosmos, the universe,
depend on others in the universe.

Hence people for generations talk of
Cosmic rays,
Cosmic energy,
Cosmic awareness,
Cosmic perception,
Cosmic consciousness,
and
hence
always look up to
the cosmos
for everything
when in trouble.

32   *Ko Paandu*

COSMOS:

When we gaze at the sky in the night, not all the stars but so
many within the limitation of the human eyes are visible to
us. Humans are attached to the nature and hence everyone is
attracted to the events of the nature, the atmospheric states,
the rain, the wind, and the conditions what they bring. The
sky and the space beyond our view are the ones that created the
eagerness for the human race to search more and more in moon
and the planets and even beyond the solar system. The night
is cool or warm based on the place where from the individual
looks at, warm countries or cold places and hence there is a
tendency to stay outdoors and an eagerness to look at the sky.
The sky too is attractive with its stars and moon. The day sky
with shining sun is attractive in cold countries and is not that
attractive in hot counties due to the shining sun. Even day sky
becomes attractive when it creates a spectacle with thunder
and lightning, when the sky shows its colors by its clouds in
the background of the sun and the horizon. We look outside
when the ramblings from inner voice due to problems craving
for solutions and when we need to feel free from the interior
troubles. The energy of the sun, moon, planets and the stars
has effect on us and their energy exists in us too. It is not only
in the human body, animals and the roots of the plants but
in every cell and the elements on the earth and elsewhere in
space. The reason being all elements in the universe are part
of one close-knit family.

Moon revolves on its own and comes around the earth. Same
way earth rotates about itself and comes around the sun. The
sun also rotates on its own and comes around the Milky Way
Galaxy. The galaxy too does rotate itself and the process is
endless in time and unlimited in space. To come down to
the molecules, atoms and the atomic particles, they also have
rotations. How come everything rotates and is still stable.
The reason is the existence of the magnetic field and gravity

throughout the objects in space from electron to the stars and other large objects in the cosmos. The stability is like a bicycle's stability, only so long as its wheels rotate and it is moving. The magnetic field and electric filed are partners in establishing the links of bodies of the cosmic space.

All the objects in this universe have their own magnetic axis, around which they revolve. The living cells at the microscopic level also have magnetic field with positive and negative polarisations.

Magnetic force and electricity are active partners. A current flow through a metallic wire conductor can produce a magnetic field. Also a conductor movement in a magnetic field can produce a current. No interaction between magnetic and electric fields when they are static. When a metallic wire, which is a current conductor, cuts a magnetic field, electrical current is produced and flows in the wire. This equals to a generator of electricity. Same way when a wire with current flow under a magnetic field would move the wire akin to a motor. This is the active and dynamic effect of the two basic natural forces that is part of every object in the universe from the smallest atomic particle, electron, to the biggest object in space. The magnetic field due to electrical is called electromagnetic fields and this field imparts electromagnetic

What is Electron?

In electricity we get power by movement of electrons. Everything in the world is made up of atoms. Many atoms combine to make a molecule. Different Molecules make a cell and cells constitute the body of living animal or human being.

Every element has the centre core called nucleus and electrons circling around the nucleus. Electrons are free to jump and get away if any force acts on them. Bonding between atoms and molecules are due to electrons.

Chemistry is a subject which deals with bonding of electrons with other elements or molecules to form different molecules and compounds.

force. In static conditions magnets have magnetic field and a voltage without current flow has electric field (Robert O. Becker, 1998)

The electrical and magnetic forces are the reason for the energy in the human cells. The atmosphere gives us the energy in the form electrically charged ions. That is the energy which gives the cells the life force. The old societies are deep in the analysis of human nature and have names for life force. The life force in China is called *'chi (qi)'*, in India it is called as *'prana'*, Japanese call as *'ki'*, Greeks call *'pneuma'*, Arabic *'ruh'* and *'ruach'* in Hebrew.

Cosmos is beyond earth and solar system. In simple words the particle that enters earth's atmosphere from cosmic outer space is called cosmic rays.

Charged ions –Electrons:

Cosmic rays emanate from space from the objects in the universe and enter into every object in space. One of the cosmic objects, earth, utilise the particles from space and by natural process ionisation happens in the atmosphere. Any particle from space that enters into earth atmosphere has to interact with earth's atmospheric air. Air has the elements, consisting of electrons around them. During interaction and collision of the particles from cosmos with the components of atmosphere, electrons from elements of air get stripped and knocked out. During this process the particles split and get scattered and many elements from the molecules of air get stripped producing both POSITIVE and NEGATIVE ions in the atmosphere. These ionic particles are due to the absence of electrons or extra electrons. Even when the man-made dead satellites enter into the atmosphere they are burnt due to the friction and the high speed and interactive force at which objects transit through the atmosphere.

Both positive and negative ions exist in atmosphere in certain proportions. The negative ions that are part of part of air become part of our breathing and part of every biological life on earth and is called cosmic energy.

This Negative ion called NEGION and positive ion is called POSION. Negative ion is Anion and Positive ion is Cation in scientific terminology. Understanding the simple structure of an atom (see Fig.1) will help us to know the formation of ions.

The same is applicable to the molecules, which are the combination of many types of atoms. In simple terms pure copper is formation of copper atoms in full. Pure gold is formed by only atoms of gold.

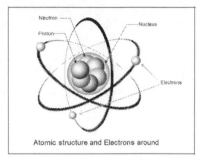

Atomic structure and Electrons around

Fig. 1

Water is a molecule formed by hydrogen and oxygen atoms. One molecule of water is formed by two atoms of hydrogen and one of oxygen. Both Hydrogen and oxygen are gases and they combine to form liquid, the water. This way in nature we have atoms and molecules, the combination of atoms.

ATOM:

An atom has a core and its surroundings. Atom consists of neutrons, protons and electrons. Core is called nucleus which contains neutron and proton. The electrons are circling around the nucleus. Proton is positively charged and electron is negatively charged. Neutron is charge free. Every atom has equal number of protons and electrons. The number of neutrons in most of the atoms are normally equal or higher in number than the protons.

Let us study in simple terms from the basic atom how the ions are formed. As an example the structure of copper atom is explained. A copper atom has 29 protons and 35 neutrons in the nucleus and 29 electrons around the nucleus. The character of atom as copper is defined by the number of protons only and that is called the Atomic number. Each atom has its own atomic number. For example atomic number of gold is 79 and has 79 protons and 119 neutrons at the nucleus.

Water has two hydrogen atoms (Atomic number of hydrogen is 1 with only one proton in its nucleus without any proton and one electron around) and one oxygen atom (Atomic number oxygen is 8 with 8 protons and 8 neutrons in its nucleus and 8 electrons around).

Charge of an Electron:

One Negative ion has a charge of 1 EV(Electron Volt) and equals to $1.60217657 \times 10^{-19}$ coulombs. EV is a basic unit to measure small charges. One Coulomb equals 6.3×10^{18} EV. ie 1 Coulomb=63,000,000,000,000,000,000 EV

3600 Coulomb is the capacity of 1000 mAH (milli Ampere Hour) AA or AAA size chargeable cell, which have capacity from 500 to 3000 mAH.
You can imagine how small an EV is.

Combined weight of protons, neutrons and electrons decide the weight of an atom and that way weight of that metal or gas. Two hydrogen atoms and one oxygen atoms forms water and the weight of water is 1 gm/cc. Weight of gold is 19.3 gm/cc (grams per cubic centimetre).

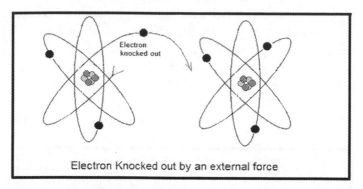

Electron
knocked out

Electron Knocked out by an external force

Fig. 2

Neutral state of an Atom:

A normal atom (see Fig.1) remains neutral when the number of protons and electrons are same. The value of the charge of an electron is same as that of proton. When an atom in a molecule or compound of molecules combine with atom of another molecule sharing the electrons between them, a strong bonding is created and the combination becomes another molecule. The resulting molecule has no free electrons. With equal number of both the protons and electrons the charge gets neutralised in an atom. The stability in electronic charge of an atom or molecule means the atom never gets disturbed. A molecule or atom may combine with another atom or molecule to form a new molecule. Yet no ionic charge is created. The atoms or molecules share the electrons between them. When an electron or electrons in an atom is attracted to another atom and combine, a molecule is formed and this is called as chemical process and the elements stay together and the new molecule is also stable. At the same time when an electron is freed from an atom (see Fig.2), a way of knock out, gets out and joins and stays with another atom. The atom which loses the electron loses a charge equivalent to the charge of an electron. By this the loser or the electron donor gets positively charged.

The atom which receives or acquires an electron becomes negatively charged (see Fig.3). The charge of atoms, loser and gainer has charge equal to the charge of an electron. These negions may be atoms or molecules or particles with a combination of so many molecules. These negions are small molecules and free to wander in air. It may get attracted to positively charged particles and particles will get neutralised.

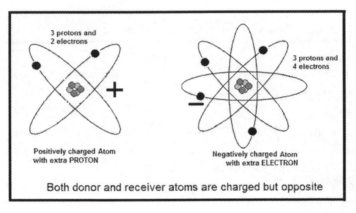

Fig. 3

We have ionised particles with positive and negative charges in atmosphere. The atmosphere consists of air which contains oxygen, nitrogen, carbon di-oxide and so many other gases.

Our life depends very much on the atmosphere and hence we have to care about it. The atmosphere gets graded in high and low in various parameters when we go up and up. The atmosphere extends only up to certain height over the earth's surface and beyond that the air is absent. There are different layers (Table-2) of the atmosphere, categorised, based on its state and conditions of temperature, temperature gradient, air density and air contents.

Table-2 Atmospheric layers

Troposphere	0 to 12 kms	0 to 7 miles
Stratosphere (also ozone layer)	12 to 50 kms	7 to 31 miles
Mesosphere	50 to 80 kms	31 to 50 miles
Thermosphere (includes Ionosphere)	80 to 700 kms	50 to 440 miles
Exosphere	700 to 10,000 kms	440 to 6,200 miles

The layer troposphere extends from surface of the earth to 12 km (0 to 7 miles). The distance of the troposphere from the earth varies from poles to equator. The layer extends up to 8 kms (Kilometres) at poles. Troposphere is the layer for the life on earth and the air is denser and contains 75% of the mass of the whole atmosphere. World's weather takes place only in this region. The temperature decreases to a level of -60°C at 12 kms. Temperature increases in Stratosphere by increasing altitude and reaches from 60°C to 0°C. The temperature rise is due to the absorption of UV rays from the sun. This layer has no air turbulence like troposphere and free of clouds.

Mesosphere is the third layer. By increase of the altitude the temperature decreases to -100°C. This is the coldest of the layers of the atmosphere. This is the layer where the meteors burn when they enter into atmosphere and shooting stars seen.

Thermosphere is the hot region with low air density. The sun heats up the atmosphere raising the temperature to 1000°C. Due to sun's high impact with low air density ionisation takes place in this region.

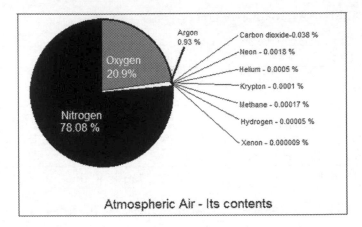

Fig.4

What do we have in this atmosphere for us to survive and also keep the plants and animals energetic apart from just surviving?

Air contains primarily oxygen as a fuel for energy production for life on earth. Major constituents of dry air are (Fig-4) Nitrogen, Argon, Neon, Helium, Krypton and Xenon and they are inert gases. Inert means that there is no chemical reaction with other elements. Apart from the above mentioned gases, atmospheric air is polluted with so many gases from chemical and other manmade industries. Oxygen and Carbon-dioxide play a major role to feed energy to the living.

The atmosphere feeds us with cosmic energy as negative ions. With these charges in space our life is intermingled and influenced by the balanced nature of both Positive and negative ions.

The Nitrogen is our DNA,
the calcium is our teeth,
the iron is our blood,
the carbon in our apple pies were made
in the interiors of collapsing stars.
We are made of star stuff.

-Carl Sagon-

4

Posions and Negions

Life has ups and downs
Our moods are elated and happy on the rise
and dips to sadness on the fall.

But

what goes up will have to come down.
Gain and loss are relative
Anything that is closing will also open
Earning is only to spend.
We may fall and get up and may fall again.
There is no tall if no short exists.
Sadness is due to absence of Enjoyment
Day looks bright because of darkness at night
Light shines when surrounding is dark.

Life sails smooth on even keel
only when
we learn to accept both sides with equipoise

Positive and Negative ions in everyday life:

Life without problems may not be interesting. Like a coin, every subject and event in the world has two sides and even thinking in life has another side and some events may have many sides. The two sided events coexist and cannot be separated. Example is the symbol called Taijitu (see Fig.5) for Yin Yang. Yang represents the bright, day, male etc. as Yin represents dark, night, female etc. One is mingled with the other. To be happy in life, all depends

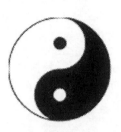

Taijitsu

Fig. 5

on how we utilise the both sides of everything. While we utilise the sun, its brightness and spend more time working in the day, we take rest with few hours of the night with darkness. We optimise and utilise both. We don't reject the other side and also one cannot reject even if one does not like it. If one reject it then nothing exists for that person and the life is unbalanced. There cannot be a coin with just one side.

We have to live with both positive and negative of everything, but with a balance. Living with the atmosphere of both positive and negative ions is the life. The word Positive and negative has nothing to do with positive benefits and negative effects over the persons. They are just identified as positively charged and negatively charged ions. The negative ions have beneficial effects for human health over the positive ions. Negions make our mind calm, tranquil and relaxed. The positive ions too help to benefit in case of germination of seeds.

Cosmic and Sources of ions:

Cosmic space is bombarded with cosmic rays and in turn creates negative ions. Apart from large amount of negative ions due to cosmic rays, there exist various sources for the positively charged ions and particles. Many manmade industries release various gases with ionised particles as a waste product. All type of gases released to the environment from industries and automobiles are waste products. Most of these from the industries are positively charged particles. The bad *Witches* winds create more positively charged dust particles in air. The dust and pollen from trees are another source of positive ions.

Nature creates ions in different ways. Below are the main sources for the positive ions and negative ions.

- Cosmic rays or cosmic particles
- Sun and Ultra violet rays in sunlight.
- Earth's radioactivity
- Natural radioactivity in rocks.
- The breaking of water droplets in waterfalls, sea waves, surfing and rain.
- Electrical discharge during lightning.
- Friction due to air movement - winds and turbulence in the atmosphere

Cosmic Particles:

The Particles from space, the primary cosmic particles, when they enter into the earth's atmosphere, have different actions in different layers of atmospheric air. Cosmic rays are mainly of high energy protons of hydrogen nuclei, alpha particles, (two protons and two neutrons like helium atom but without electrons) few heavier atoms and smaller amount of electrons.

The Cosmic rays travel through space at very high speed near to the speed of light. Also high energy packets known as photons, from space, travel at speed of light. All the cosmic particles collide first at the atmospheric layer, thermosphere. The energy of the primary cosmic particle is so high it creates a shower of charged particles when it collides with components of air. The cosmic particles travel further with reduced energy and are called secondary cosmic particles. Some cosmic particles reach earth without much hindrance but with reduced speed after many collisions.

What exactly happens when cosmic particles collide in thermosphere and further? The particles hit the molecules of nitrogen, oxygen and carbon dioxide in air and electrons are knocked out (Fig-2). More air ionisation takes place in Stratosphere

Energy of Cosmic particle and electron:

Energy of a cosmic ray is as high as 10 GeV (10,000,000,000 eV). Compare Energy an electron which is 1 eV. The energy of cosmic ray gets degraded when it reaches the earth's surface and few may enter into earth's surface with high energy.

Think of the high energy cosmic particles that will affect the astronauts of the space mission.

and Troposphere which is up to the level of 50 kms (30 Miles) from earth's surface. The electron knocked out from molecules of air may be one or more. The molecules that lose the electrons are now positively charged. The free electrons in air combine with the other neutral molecules of nitrogen, oxygen and carbon dioxide and form negatively charged particles. Whenever more than one electron is knocked out from one molecule, one posion is created but more electrons are released. They join with other molecules creating more negions. By this way negions are more in number than Posions. Most of the electrons join with oxygen, the lighter of all active elements in air.

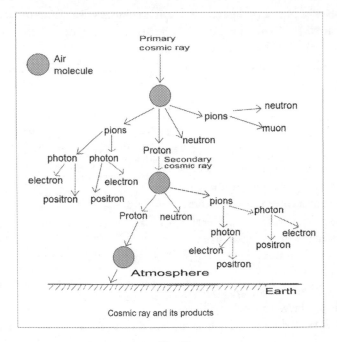

Fig.6

At the same time the negative ions combine with positively charged dust and make a clean atmosphere. One of the beneficial functions of cosmic energy is the cleaning of atmospheric air. The ionisation has lot more effect on global temperature and the climate, air precipitation, cloud formation, creation of aerosols, ozone and electrical properties of the atmosphere including lightning.

Atmosphere is the protection for the life on earth. The atmosphere, not only absorbs most of the infrared and ultraviolet rays, but also curtails the effect of high energy cosmic rays. The high-energy particles of the so-called primary cosmic ray will collide with the oxygen or nitrogen atoms in the atmosphere and then become secondary particles.

These secondary particles have sufficient energy to produce the next generation particles (see Fig.6). By successive transformations, a large cluster of particles of both ionic charges are produced. However, most of these particles get absorbed or decayed in the atmosphere. Very few cosmic particles reach the Earth's surface. The energies of the particles that hit the surface of the Earth are very low when it approaches the earth's surface. By these acts harmful effects of high energy cosmic particles are reduced. This is the way the atmosphere acts like an umbrella to protect the bioactivity.

What is the source of Cosmic particles in space? Baade and Zwicky suggested in 1934 that the cosmic rays originate from supernovae. In 1948 H.W. Babcock suggested that magnetic variable stars could be a source of cosmic rays. Y. Sekido and his colleagues suggested in 1951 that cosmic rays emanate from the Crab Nebula. Research is still in progress with acceptance and contradictions by the suggestions of the scientists. Suggestions of the sources for cosmic rays include supernovae, active galactic nuclei, quasars, and gamma-ray bursts (Walter, 2012)

Isotopes and Nuclear energy rays:

Isotopes of an atom have same physical and chemical properties. It has same number of protons and electrons, but different no of neutrons. When the no of neutrons are high compared to a stable atom there is instability.

This unstable condition releases energy in form of radiation. This atom is called radioactive. By releasing energy the unstable atom tries to get stable. There are three types of energy rays coming out of the nucleus and is called alpha, beta or gamma. One or more type of rays is released from an isotope. These rays interact with other elements and knocks out electrons creating both positive and negative ions.

One of the isotopes of an element is the source for radiation in cancer treatment

Sun's energy:

Solar wind consists mostly of high energy electrons and protons. The high energy particles when they interact with air more electrons are knocked out creating more negions. High energy packet, photon, from sun acts to knock out electrons. Ionisation of air molecules occurs in ionosphere due to Ultraviolet rays of the sun. Ionosphere is the upper atmosphere region as part of the thermosphere, 80 kms (50 miles) from earth's surface extending to 700 kms (440 miles). Sun's energy is strong and in this region the ultraviolet rays breaks the molecules of air creating ionised particles.

Earth's radioactivity:

A meagre amount of ions are formed from the earth's radioactivity. Earth has many minerals and natural elements, which has isotopes. These isotopes (see text box) are radioactive. These radioactive elements ionise the atmosphere by adding more negative ions out of its action on surface of the earth. Modern society by its concrete structures reduces the flow of radiation and obstructs the path for the release of ions into atmospheric air.

Natural radioactivity in rocks:

This is similar to earth's radioactivity but in open space from the isotopes of mineral elements from mines and rocks. Radon, in gas form, is also another source of ions which occurs naturally during the decay of thorium and uranium.

Waterfalls, sea waves, surfing and rain:

We enjoy the waterfalls, water fountains and bathroom showers. When air passes through water or air, it has interaction with water molecules and produces more negions than posions.

This can be felt near the water waves hitting the sea shore. The surfers enjoy the ride due to the comfortable sensation it creates. Light air flow in drizzling and during heavy rain causes a cool, soothing and relaxing sensation. Waterfalls create freshness of vegetation. Just imagine the places people want to visit and roam around. Those are the places with more negative ions available that creates a relaxed mind.

Lightning causes ionisation:

Why lightning? The positively charged clouds get attracted by the earth. The reason is that the earth is negatively charged. The clouds are of different categories, charged positive or negative or without any charge. When the positively charged clouds are close to the earth there is attraction between positive cloud and negative earth. Same way the joining of the clouds of opposite charges in the sky is the lightning above our head or far away in the horizon. The tallest building or a tree attracts the positive cloud, which makes a heavy current flow that makes an arc which is lightning and sound out of it is the thunder. The lightning is the flash of arcing due to the high current discharge. This is like an electrical short circuit with a heavy current. In the house a short circuit current of 10 amps opens the breaker. Lightning short circuits are of the order of 5,000 to 50,000 amps in 0.2 seconds. Air is ionised before lightning strikes. After the electrical discharge during lightning most of the ions get neutralised. Some charged particles remain in atmosphere. The rain brings down the heavy particles. That is the reason for the high positive ions during lightning and then high negative ions compared to positive ions during rain.

> **Current during Lightning:**
>
> 100 watts light bulb draws around 1 amp (110V) or 0.5 amps (220V). Lightning causes a current flow of 5000 Amps just for few seconds. That show the strength of the cloud and how much charge is accumulated in the cloud.

In olden days many tall buildings got demolished during rainy season by lightning. People believed the destruction was due to ire of gods and a punishment for some of the misdeeds of the people. Some building stayed stable even after many lightning strikes. Later it was found that the structures, uniform in construction in verticality stayed without lightning strikes. A building with sharp tips on top of the structure helped the stability. By this experience, metallic polls or metallic tips were installed and this design continued in churches and temples. The metallic tips and strips create a short circuiting path with the ground, avoiding the current passing through the building and damaging it.

Winds and turbulences in the atmosphere:

When dry air moves along the land plains it takes the dust, pollens and every positively charged particle along with it. The dry air from the plains when hits the mountain surface it creates a rubbing action and creates ions both positive and negative. The negative ions produced are less and also most of the negative ions produced are consumed by the positively charged dust and dust is deposited along its way in land, houses, etc. Many such winds are explained in earlier chapters.

The generation of negative ions in its concentration has a closer relation with wind speed, water, plants and humidity of air. The most important factor is water and then the wind. Temperature of air has less significance.

History of observations and findings of ionic charges:

For centuries people knew that the air has various effects on the persons based on the climates not only due to temperature and moisture but also something other than that. Hippocrates, in 5th century, observed "northern winds occasion disorder and sickness".

In 1748, Jean Antoine Nollet, a French clergyman and physicist invented one of the first electrometers, the electroscope, which detected the presence of electric charge by using electrostatic attraction and repulsion. He had done an experiment by planting mustard seeds in two pots. Using an electrostatic generator he passed the positive charges to one pot and nothing to the second pot. After about a week all the seeds planted in the first pot sprouted and shown their growth by few millimetres where as the second pot showed very little progress compared to the first pot.

In late 18th century, Giuseppe Toaldo, who was a priest, was appointed to the chair of astronomy in the University of Padua. Toaldo paid great attention to the study of atmospheric electricity. He became a famous physicist and professor. He observed that plant growth has some link with the electricity that exists in air as static electricity. He observed that the plants growing next to a lightning rod grew almost ten times taller than identical plants just a few meters away. Based on the views of Benjamin Franklin of US, he promoted the erection of lightning rods, as a preventive and protective action. By his pressure, lightning conductors were installed to protect the tall structures on Siena Cathedral, on the tower of St. Mark's in Venice. Venetian navy also adopted his method to install lightning arresters on ships.

In 1780 Abbe Bertholon of France observed some electrical state of air causes changes in people's health. He noticed that vegetables grew an extraordinary size when water was electrified by electrostatic generator and poured on them. Also he invented a unit to collect atmospheric electricity using an antenna and passed the ionized air on to plants and named the unit as "electro-vegeto-meter".

Even though many persons have proved that static electricity has its say over the plant growth and also documented and demonstrated, the understanding of the reasons was not easy. No one was able to explain how it happens.

During 1899, German physicists Julius Elster and Hans Friedrich Geitel, proved that electrostatic fields were based upon the existence of electrically charged particles called ions. In order to prove this, experiments were conducted by a team at the Air Ion Laboratory of the University of California. By passing electrically charged particles over the plants, it was proved that the growth rates of the plants are high and the ions have a physiological effect on the plants.

In 1901 PeterCzermak of Germany suggested that the air ions in the atmosphere may cause these health problems during the winds Sharav of Israel, Mistrel of France, Santa Ana of California. Until then scientists believed that the air is being ionised by earth's radiation. A German scientist Victor Hess raised a balloon to a height of 5000 metres and in doing so found that the radiation increased with increase of altitude. That radiation at high altitude up was named as cosmic rays. His research on cosmic rays earned him a Nobel Prize.

Dr. Clarence W. Hansell of RCA Laboratories was the first to find out that ions could also have an impact on the state of mind of individuals. His observation came on a day in 1932, when he noticed a change of mood in a wild way of a colleague working near an electrostatic generator. This incident made Dr Hansell to monitor his colleague continuously. He found on another day that his colleague was cheerful and happy when the generator was made to produce negative ions. Subsequent tests proved the depression and irritability was when the machine was producing positive ions. Dr. Hansell's observations widened and started noticing the effects of atmospheric ions over individuals.

During and after 1933 serious experiments started by Albert P. Krueger, Bio-meteorologist and Professor Emeritus at the University of California and Russian scientist A.L. Tchijewsky. They reported that the growth of some bacteria is inhibited when air has high content of negative ions.

Serotonin and positive ions:

During late 1950's research by Dr. Albert Krueger proved that a small amount of negative ions could kill all types of bacteria that caused colds, influenza and respiratory infections. He then tried with large group of mice with various concentrations of ions. During his experiments, he found over production of Serotonin when the mice were subjected to positive ions leading to hyperactivity, exhaustion, anxiety and depression. Same group with negative ions introduced after stopping the positive ions, created calmness among them with serotonin reduced. This research had uncovered the mechanism fundamental to the altering moods by altering the types of ionized air. He found a reliable data that there happens a significant and consistent reduction in blood levels of serotonin when the mice were exposed to air with negative ions of 400,000 per cc. The hypothesis, he concluded was that the high dose of positive ions increase the serotonin levels and the high negative ions stimulate the action of speeding up the metabolic removal of serotonin.

Serotonin is an important chemical molecule produced in the body and is popularly thought to be a contributor to the feelings of well-being and happiness. It also plays a major role in plants and animals. Serotonin plays a major role in the human central nervous system, such as depression, mood, perception, anger, aggression, behaviour, anxiety disorder, social phobia, memory, sexual behaviour, appetite, and sleep. In addition, serotonin has important functions outside the central nervous system, including the regulation of energy balance and food intake and activities of gastrointestinal, endocrine function, cardiovascular and pulmonary physiology. Serotonin is connected with several human diseases like depression, schizophrenia, migraine, hypertension and eating disorders.

It was found that the serotonin in the brain is a factor representing positive ion levels. Negative ions help to increase the mental activity by diminishing the serotonin levels. Patients who are affected by positive ions go to a state of depression and bad moods. They are treated with medicines of the type of serotonin blockers. The medical field have contradictions in increased serotonin levels due to the reason not clear whether serotonin causes the mental depression or the mental depression causes increase of serotonin. The subject of serotonin and its effects are still in debate (Blenau, 2015).

To substantiate Dr. Krueger's findings Dr. Felix G. Sulman, head of the department of Applied Pharmacology at Hebrew University in Jerusalem discovered the primary cause behind the unpleasant symptoms experienced by people in the desert region during the period of poison winds. He could link the people's moods during the winds of Sharav to the winds of Sirrocco in Italy, *Foehn* in Central Europe, and the Santa Ana in California (Soyka, 1991).

Full moon and positive ions:

The moon reflects the sun light to its maximum during full moon. The surface of the moon has negative ions like the surface of the earth. The photons from the sun get reflected by the moon without much angle deviation and hence energetic. This negative charge of the moon by the photonic effect towards earth repels the outer layer of earth's ionosphere which is a field of negative ions. By this way the ionosphere is pushed close to the surface of the earth. This creates high population of positive ions compared to the existing negative ions. The full moon effect is due the increased positive ions.

Health during a *Foehn* wind:

In a 1980 study Dr Felix Gad Sulman collected samples of urine from 1000 volunteers regularly just before the arrival of storm of *Foehn* wind and normal weather conditions. Compared to normal weather conditions the samples taken just before the *Foehn* wind showed in analysis an increased production of serotonin. He concluded that the high concentration of positive ions, carried by these winds would stimulate an increase in production of serotonin and histamine in their bodies, causing allergies, migraines, difficulty in breathing, irritability, and anxiety. Also the samples were analysed for hormone levels, adrenaline etc. The production of adrenaline initially induces a state of euphoria and hyperactivity. Hyperthyroidism was also associated with the increased positive ion conditions. Although serotonin is extremely crucial to the functioning of our bodies, he concluded that these individuals, who are weather sensitive, produce too much serotonin during the bad winds. They were affected by their own serotonin. He thus coined the term "Serotonin Irritation Syndrome."

Dr. Werner Becker, a professor in the department of clinical neurosciences at the University of Calgary, in Alberta studied for two years, keeping record of health conditions of many patients during pre-Chinook, Chinook and non-Chinook days. Out of 75 patients 32 were likely to have migraines during the Chinook. Dr Coleman and Becker said that weather was the main migraine trigger. Chinook is a *Witches'* wind in which positive ions are in a higher level.

Cosmic rays in the Earth's atmosphere:

Solar Energy into atmosphere of the earth is around thousand million times that of energy by Cosmic rays. Hence only solar system was believed to have influence on the earth's atmosphere. However Russian scientists Ermakov and Komozokov did measurements and confirmed that ion production at the lower atmosphere due to cosmic rays is very high. Hence cosmic rays have major part in atmospheric electric current, cloud formation, thunder cloud formation, lightning production, etc (Ermakov, 1992).

The secondary rays, after losing much of its energy in the higher layer of atmosphere enter troposphere and stratosphere, producing ultra-fine aerosols. These aerosol layers have also significant effect on the atmosphere of the earth in heat balance. The ionised clouds reflect the solar light upward and earth's thermal radiation downward making the thermal balance. Recombination occurs in all of the ionisation regions always because of the presence of free positive ions and negative ions at the same place. The recombination is very low at high altitude due to high energy and high speed. At lower layer of atmosphere the recombination is high because of its slow speed of ions and big size ion particles. Particle density is also high at low altitudes (Siingh, Devendraa- 2010).

> **2250 ions in one cc :**
>
> One cc (cubic centimetre) of air contains 2.7×10^{19} molecules.
>
> 2250 ions out of this quantity is nothing compared to the total number of molecules.
>
> 1250 positively charged particles with 1000 negatively charged particlesin air is normal condition. Bad environments increase the posions to higher ratio to that of the negions from 5:4 to 12:4. 1250 to 2400 posions in proportion with 1000 to 2000 negions per cc in the ratio of around 5:4 is the best atmosphere for a normal individual.

Cosmic rays play an important role in ionisation of the atmosphere than the sun's rays. Ionisation of the region above the clouds has the impact of the charges ionising the particles of the cloud. The interesting chain of reactions is that the ionized particles charge the clouds, clouds cause lightning and lightning again produces charged particles of both types.

Approaching rain with lightning and thunder:

Hair raising feeling happens during lightning and thunder due to the presence of high positive ions. Also when clouds of positive ions are close to earth and near us, elated feeling will arise with euphoria. A thunder heard immediately after a flash of lightning means the cloud collisions occurred very near. More time gaps between light and sound is because of far away clouds. The time difference is due to the long travel of high speed of light and low speed of sound. By the time drizzling starts, the elated feeling dies down, and the rain brings a chilly feeling owing to the negative ions.

Agriculture - Seeding and planting:

Investigators have found that plants have some kind of sensitivity to the negative ions and positive ions. Planting the trees and many of the crops, as per Old Farmer's Almanac, around the time of full moon makes them grow better. This early growth also gives better yields later. Vegetables like lettuce, tomatoes, carrots etc. planted during the full moon time grows faster and healthier than those planted in the other days. Scientists reason that the positive ions are more during this time of full moon and these ions play an important role in water absorption by the plants from the roots. Positive ions play a role in sub soil level for the sprouting and inner core part of the plant where as negative ions helps in the outer layer of the plant.

Farmers in South Indian Tamilnadu sow the seeds at the last few days of the month of *Aadi*. The *Aadi* wind creates an abundance of positive ions during the month. Seeding is done on the last days of the month and thus positive ion helps the seed to germinate. Subsequently the monsoon rain takes care of the plants like Raagi, millet, Choalam, Varagu, Saamai etc. of the south Indian dry land varieties.

Ion Comfort with Posion versus Negion:

As already explained in the previous chapter comfort of human being is when both positive ions and negative ions are present in a certain proportion. 5:4 is the best ratio of positive and negative ions. For 5 posions, 4 negions are normal and comfortable. Every individual has different requirement of ions. Because of these reasons not all people are affected during the increased posion levels. Some unventilated areas increase the posions to 4 times of negions like in closed rooms, cars with doors closed, room air-conditioners with locally circulated air, Industrial areas with dust and during approaching storm.

Out of both ions, negative ions what we call COSMIC ENERGY enables to maintain a balance with the positive ions and plays an important role in our health.

"The universal law is that knowledge and
awareness that all living things - all life -
has within it the vitality and strength
to gather from itself
all things necessary
for its growth and function"

-from the book, 'Who in fact you really are'-

5

Cosmic Energy in Health

We have.
But
we are not using what we have,
because
we do not know that we have.

What we require is near us.
But we are always searching for
something
that is far away.

What is close to us is cheap and
What we are after may be costly.

We are trying for costly solutions
for simple problems.

The Solution is in us.
We need a simple key to solve
our problem
and
we should know how to use the key.

All energy is Up on Tops and in Tips:

An individual, when he is on the top of a building, feels elated. There is also an interest to walk up the stairs or go by elevators to have a feel of the building top. Why? Children want to climb the trees. Even with all risks, the interest is to climb up and up. Reaching the tree top is more interesting and the enthusiasm the tree top creates is by imparting the energy to the climber. There is

> **Charged Metal ball:**
> A smooth metal ball of a ball bearing will not have a tip or burr. If that metal ball with uniform surface is carrying a charge, all the charges will be spread uniformly on its surface with equal surface distribution.
>
> If a needle is charged, all charges will reside at the tip of the needle.

enjoyment too when sitting under the branches of the tree. Tree houses are another way of invitation by the tree to feed energy to the sleepers. There is something very subtle that creates an interest in them to go up the tree. When people climb the hills or mountains, the feeling of tiredness is less and nullified by the interest in climbing. Reason for this entire inner urge to climb is the presence of the cosmic energy.

The earth is a negatively charged mass. Characteristic of any charged particle is to reside in the tip of the body. Every tip of an object on earth's surface will be having a high negative charge. In case of non-uniform body, building, trees, hills or mountains, the tips are the attraction for the charges. Earth is negatively charged and these negative ions of the earth always tend to be concentrated more at the top with its attraction to the clouds of opposite charge. When the positively charged clouds come close to earth, the negatively charged earth shows its face on the top of hills, trees and tall buildings. The atmosphere above has both positive and negative charges. Always there is hide and seek of the earth and atmosphere for us to enjoy and suffer with thunder and lightning.

What way negions help with its presence on top of the hill or tree tops? Many temples, churches and pagodas built over the hills have more attraction. The holy places are built on hill tops and by reaching the pilgrims return with a feeling of relaxed mind and that feeling stays in their mind and re-energizes them for a long time. Also that experience motivates them to make another visit to that sacred place. Even though the climbing is difficult, one feels fresh on reaching the top. This is the reason why many holy places on hill-tops have an attraction. An individual gets energy without his knowledge. There is a pleasant feeling one gets after the visit to the place, but does not know what it is or how to describe it.

The earth is the biggest negatively charged mass. Touching the ground with bare foot and hands makes one feel contented. That is the reason for most passengers to get down from a bus during a brief halt en route and walk on the ground. The land surface imparts a sense of relief from the stress induced by travel. Same way kids have interest to play in the mud, which really gives lot of energy to them. It is not the clay with which they wish to play, it is the soil of the earth with which they like to play, however messy it is.

Atmosphere by way of air gives us oxygen to give energy to have power for the living cells to keep the bio system alive. To be energetic and dynamic? Something else is needed to keep the mind energetic and to act. That is the negative ions, which is part of air, that is working its magic on us without our self knowing or realising what it is.

History of Research in Negative ions:

Human race have been experiencing the elated, excited, energizing and refreshing effects of negative ions in different forms from rain, breeze, waterfalls, water showers for thousands of years. Experience by those interested in various subjects such as the logic, hypothesis and formulae based on mathematics has taken the shape of science. Those who created equations have become scientists. Wherever the observation of people cannot be scaled to the measurable values, they cannot be introduced in mathematics. They still lie as observations and the observers are naturalists and are continuously trying to fit into the present day science. They did not know the reason why the actions of natural events cannot be equated to measurable values in science. However they just enjoy nature and talk about cosmos. Scientists whoever wants to links natural events with hypothesis, go only with uncertainties, probabilities and statistical way.

Keen observations by people who live in harmony with nature and their little knowledge of modern day science make them to link various day-to-day observations and subjects to improve their life. Electricity is one of such subjects which could be linked to the growth of plants by some botanists and plant science enthusiasts.

Even before the west entered into the science arena, easterners have started using methods to utilize the energy of the nature for their health improvement and as medicinal power. The olden methods to preserve the health are followed through generations as learned from elders and are continuing even now.

Cosmic energy in Pyramid:

In the 1930s, Antoine M. Bovis, a Frenchman observed that a dead cat in the Great Pyramid did not decompose. The animal apparently wandered into the King's Chamber and perished before finding an exit route. The cat's body dried out, although the air in the King's Chamber is always humid. Egyptologists have found well preserved grain in tombs that was thousands of years old. Normally grains in modern silos keep no longer than four years. The preservation of organic material in pyramids has received a lot of attention. Bovis had returned to France with the mystery of the mummified cats still lingering in his mind.

Bovis's observation gave rise to the idea of *'pyramid power'*, which preserves organic matter. Several models made of paper, wood or other materials have been tested for desiccating organic matter. Several tests have demonstrated pyramid to be capable of preserving organic matter. The shape and direction is the key to the phenomenon popularly known as *'pyramid power'*. The lines that formed the base of the Great Pyramid ran due north and south on two sides and east and west on the other two. Once the pyramid structure was done and properly sized, Bovis placed the body of a dead cat on the platform, lowered his small pyramid over it, and waited to see what happened. Several weeks later, an odd change came over the animal's corpse. Instead of decaying and drawing flies as Bovis expected, it had withered, dried up, and became a mummy. Like the dead animals he had seen in the King's Chamber of the great pyramid, it did not decay and it did not smell foul. No scientist he talked to could explain this strange transformation.

Pyramid could sharpen the blade:

Karl Drbal, a Czechoslovakian scientist and an electronics engineer from Prague wanted to test the energy in the pyramid. He constructed a small cardboard model of the Great Pyramid, arranged in so many ways and finally lined up in north and south directions and kept over a platform. He kept a used razor blade below the pyramid and on the platform overnight. The next morning he shaved using the blade and it seemed sharper than the morning before. Drbal, had a theory that the model pyramid acted as a kind of magnifying glass, capturing energies that fell to earth and focusing them on its interior.

He continued his experiments and filed for a patent calling his discovery the "Cheops Pyramid Razor Blade Sharpener". The officials in the Czech Patent Office laughed in his face; but, when they tested his claims, they discovered, to their amazement, that it worked exactly the way he said it would. Later Drbal went into business for himself with Patent #91304 for his pyramid blade sharpener (Boyle, 1975).

Ordinary tap water was changed overnight under the influence of the powers of a pyramid. The sprinkled water made the plants grew taller and faster. People who drank pyramid water have claimed to feel more alert and healthier. Some people had built pyramids the size of small rooms where they can sit quietly and be reenergized by the pyramid forces. As a result of sitting in these rooms, many people claim that ailments such as toothaches, headaches, and backaches disappeared, and that their thinking and concentration improved as well.

Russian scientist, Dr. A. L. Tchijewsky, tried raising mice, rats, guinea pigs, and rabbits in totally de-ionized air, clean oxygen but removing all ions. Almost all of them died within two weeks. This proved that negative ions are needed in order to utilize the oxygen in the body. Dr. D. A. Lapitsky, colleague of Tchijewsky experimented with the small animals in air completely devoid of oxygen. As they were about to die from asphyxiation he added only negative ions to the air. At which point, their respiration frequency drastically increased, as they began to sit up and run around. Ionized air is more important than the oxygen is the conclusion (Tchijewski, 1960).

Negative ions and Cell energy:

Our body is made up of various types of cells. The cell is an energy engine and millions of cell engines are required to make the body alive and act energetically. The mitochondrion in a cell is called the power house of the cell and has a fuel molecule called ATP (Adenosine TriPhosphate). Mitochondrion converts energy from food into ATP. ATP production is the basic requirement for the body cells to maintain and rectify the bad body tissues by producing new cells or repairing them. ATP production is part of respiratory activity where the energy creation in the cell happens. In the Respiratory Chain of fuel burning and energy creation, one enzyme, in the reaction, grabs the glucose molecule first. Then reacts with an oxygen molecule and absorbs the reaction energy to make ATP. Also, two electrons are removed from hydrogen atoms on molecules associated with the respiratory chain reaction and are used by these enzymes to facilitate the oxidation reaction. This process of oxidation reaction, use the reaction energy to make ATP, and the passing along of the two electrons with what is left of the glucose molecule. This continues until nothing is left of the glucose molecule and the two electrons leave in the final byproducts of the oxidation reactions. Living is just the static survival and more than that is the dynamic action. ATP is the energy for the cell to live and to act. Act means to walk, run and fight from external disease causing agents and that is the immune system to protect the cell itself. Inaction is dull and laziness and just living.

In an ideal condition all the above goes well and one enzyme always successfully passes both electrons to the next enzyme in the reaction chain and reaction chain continues. At one time so many chain reactions are in progress. Many will proceed in the chain reaction and some will falter. In reality something may go wrong and one of the enzymes may mishandle in the process of energy unbalance and may lose one of the electrons. If the reaction chain does not have both electrons, the oxidation reaction cannot occur in the next enzyme. Further ATP production cannot occur until that lost electron is replaced. Here enters the negative ion. The negatively charged oxygen molecules, which has an extra electron donates to fulfill the gap of the lost electron. This negatively charged oxygen molecule makes the enzyme to continue the process with oxidation reaction and thereby maintaining the ATP production without hindrance.

Metabolism is the process of acquiring nutrients from the blood and excreting waste out of the body, which is extremely important to the human cells. The more negative ions in the blood, the more efficient the process of the metabolism of the cell. On the contrary, the more positive ions in the blood, the slower and less efficient is the cell's metabolism. When our body is surrounded by both positive and negative ions, most of the negative ions enter by absorption through breathing and transporting to lungs and then to the blood. The negative ions, lost in the blood, add alkalinity to the blood. This makes prevention of acidification of the blood, which is caused by the loss of electrons. A shift occurs in your body's indicators of the blood acid-base balance toward alkalinity. The pH (potential of hydrogen) shifts to around 7.5 making it alkaline on the 1 to 14 pH scale (pH of water is 7 and is neutral; Reduced number in pH means increase in acidity. pH of 1 is the highest acidity).

It is an easy way through the breathing for negative ions to enter into the body and then to the cells. At the same time negions adsorbed through the skin surface also gets transferred into the body. Negatively charged molecules, mostly oxygen molecules, drift along the body surface upward toward the positive ionosphere. Positively charged ions, such as carbon dioxide molecules drifts down with attraction of the negative earth. During the movement of negions upward and posions downward these ions drift over the human body. A voltage gradient exists over the surface of the body which changes smoothly and cyclic manner. The human body creates a positive and a negative side of the body with the separating line from toe to head as vertical centre line. Even though the vertical centre line remains the same the movement of positive and negative charges change the sides. The polarity gets reversed about once in 15 to 20 minutes. If left side is positive and right is negative and 15 minutes later left becomes negative and right becomes positive. By the alternation of charges, the voltage gradient exists and the voltages on the body surface goes on changing smoothly from positive to negative and from negative to positive.

Our breathing process is automatic and intake air is inhaled in one nostril and output is through another nostril. Under normal conditions the body balances the ionisation by means of nasal cycle. Taking the breath in through the left nostril, the negatively charged ions enter. Breathe out lets out the positively charged ions through the right nostril. After about 15 to 20 minutes the process reverses taking the negatively charged ions in breathing through the right nostril and leaves positively charged ions through the left nostril. This cycle happens when the positive and negative charge polarity changes. In the Indian system of yoga, this has an important part in 'Pranayama'. The alternating breathing process is called 'Pingala naadi' and 'Ida naadi' and also called as breathing cycles - sun and moon.

The voltage gradient moves the negative ions along the skin surface and in doing so the charges are drawn into high positive voltage points in the body. The points with positive voltages are the acupuncture points in the meridian system. These acupuncture points are 361 in total and is distributed throughout the body. Each acupuncture point is around one mm in diameter. The negative ions, mostly oxygen molecules, are taken into the acupuncture points of the meridians. The charged ions enter through the capillaries and then to the cell membranes.

Negative ion in Health:

Our modern life made our homes, offices, public places and transport systems modern but away from nature. This made the environment unhealthy because of modern building materials like enclosed rooms, ventilation systems with forced air, artificial electrical lightings emitting electromagnetic radiation, synthetic industrial produces replacing natural materials and modern office gadgets like computers and mobiles with a wide range of radiating energies and waves.

Miscellaneous uses of Negative Ion generators including research:

With all comforts of modern life, the attraction of nature never leaves us alone and the environment continues to make us live on the surface of this earth. With all the advantages of negative ions one requires to be near a waterfall, water fountain, rain showers and breeze through the trees. For one to be in these environments whenever he needs may not be possible. One can now have the benefits of negative ions if a negative ion generator is plugged in the room. These generators can create the ionized atmosphere of the natural events even though they cannot match the natural sources. The generation can be made balanced with positive to negative ions. These negative ion generators helped the scientists, doctors and other researchers to experiment with people to know more about the basics of ions and their use.

Negative ion generators are used in military in the cock-pit of fighter jets and naval submarines, with closed environments. Also to have an increase in alertness and concentration, ion generators are used in normal ships. When away from earth's atmosphere and being in closed space the crew requires negions and NASA provides negative ion generators in their space shuttles.

Some dentists are now using negative ion generators to help maintain a sterile environment, neutralize toxic mercury vapour when removing old fillings, and to calm patients. Some

Las Vegas casinos get rid of tobacco odours and keep their players feel happy and alert by pumping negative ions into the air. Toyota central R&D labs found the effect of negions in improving fatigue and cognition of drivers.

Air ionization by the electronically induced formation of small air ions made significant reductions in airborne microbes, neutralization of odours, and reductions of specific volatile organic compounds. Air ionization also helped to remove the very fine particulates (Daniels, 2002).

Negions for room cleanliness:

Room air conditioners have dust collection techniques using negative ion generators. Most of the dusts in the rooms are charged particles and that too positively charged heavy particles. These charged particles will not settle down on the floor easily. Charged particles are active and having that much energy to run around and not to settle down to the floor. The technique to settle down is to have the opposite charge and neutralise the dust. The opposite charge of dust is negative ions and is generated as part of air conditioner. The negative ions thus generated are fed in the place where air from the room is sucked for filtering, cooling and recirculation. The attraction between two opposite ions makes the dust neutralised and lifeless and is filtered easily. Else filtering a charged dust is difficult as that will stick on the filters and clog the filters fast. The negative ions here serve only for the purpose of dust filter.

Negions for a healthy room:

The purpose of the ion generator is to generate negative ions to mix with the cooled air. In a room air conditioning system much of the air is re-circulated while bit of fresh air is added if required. The fresh air brings negative ions into the room to compensate the consumed ions. The return air from the room is filtered and added with outside air. Then the air is cooled and the negative ions are mixed with before diffusing the air into the room.

Vent ducts design in HVAC:

In HVAC (Heating, Ventilation and Air Conditioning) system important point to consider is to avoid generation of positive ions in the path of air circulating ducts. High speed of air, which creates a shrill noise in ducts, induces positive ions. Dr. Charles Wallah details in his book 'Ion Controversy' that the duct designs should be with smooth bends and curves for a smooth air path and should not rub with duct parts. Air conditioner manufacturers are designing new systems that increase negative ionization. The American Broadcasting Co. has equipped its new 30 storey New York City Headquarters with ion control.

Cosmic energy in Home design - FENGSHUI of China) and Vaasthu of India):

'Fengshui' and 'Vaasthu' are the systems followed in the construction of residential buildings in China and in India respectively. The concept that continues to exist for so many generations is to decide good environment in the construction of houses. Even though some specialists decide on their own methods, many of the basics existing for years are followed even today. The purpose of Fengshui and Vaasthu is to build each room in the house for good airflow carrying the cosmic energy. Hence the size of the rooms, the location of rooms for different purposes, the kitchen, the direction at which door and windows to be placed etc. are decided. Fengshui and Vaasthu are losing their values in the modern time when house is designed with available limited area. Fengshui had been designed for houses and buildings with a piece of land around in olden days taking care of the basics on terrain, the environment, wind directions, weather conditions, rain seasons and rain directions etc. Only on knowing the basics of those concepts, new requirements can be formulated.

Based on the study in a southern coastal province of China, the urban town planning team of that town planned to improve the urban ecological environment based on the concentrations of atmospheric ions that were produced by many natural and anthropogenic sources. They planned to take effective measures to increase the distribution of negative air ion concentration in urban planning and construction (Wang Wei, 2014).

Negative ions in Offices:

Based on a study by a survey team on sickness and headaches, negative ion generators were used in the computer department of Norwich Union Insurance Group headquarters. Sickness and headaches were analysed during the test period and found that the problems got reduced by 78%. This improvement in health induced the company to install the negative ion air cleaners permanently (Soyka, 1991).

Negative ions for headaches:

Windsor and Becket of U.S. experimented by giving overdoses of positive ions to sixteen volunteers for twenty minutes at a time. All of them developed dry throats, hoarse voices, headaches, and itchy or blocked noses. Five of the volunteers were tested for total breathing capacity, and found that the capacity reduced by 30 percent. After exposing all of them to negative ions for ten minutes, the breathing capacity came to maximum. What is significant here is that negative ions did not affect the amount of air breathed, but positive ions made breathing more difficult.

Negative Ions and Mental activity:

In 1969, Dr. Sulman, subjected one group of volunteers to spend some time in a room with an air flow with reduce level of negative ions and another group in the second room with high dose of negative ions. While sitting in the rooms, the persons were given word, figure and symbol tests. The score was significantly higher on these tests with those in the second room with ion-enriched condition compared to the persons of the first room. Those in the negative ion enriched room showed via EEG (ElectroEncephaloGram) a slower, stronger pulse rate of Alpha waves from the brain. Alpha wave rhythms are a measure of healthy brain's activity. A slow, strong Alpha wave pulse rate indicates healthiness, calmness, and increased alertness. The persons in the negative ion-deficient room showed signs of irritability and fatigue in addition to lower test performance (Sulman, 1974).

Negative ions in Sports:

During 1959, Minkh found, in a group of nine Russian sports students, that running endurance was increased by 260% in 32 days compared with a normal control group. This could be achieved when they were made to inhale the air mixed with 1.5 millions of negions/cc for 15 minutes daily. Considerable increase in vital capacity was observed by M.A. Vytchikova and A. Minkh with the maintenance of blood sugar and blood oxygen levels. A team of doctors, psychologists, and physicists observed and measured the performance of Olympic athletes in various conditions of negative ions levels. To improve the performance in sports, sleeping quarters of sports centres of USSR and the then East Germany were fed with negative ions even before the 1976 Olympics.

Negative ions and Asthma and other respiratory conditions:

In 1962, Dr. A. P. Wehner of United States reported that he used negative ion generators to treat over 1,000 patients suffering from various respiratory problems. The treated cases had illness of bronchial asthma, pulmonary emphysema, laryngitis, bronchitis, dry hacking cough, upper respiratory tract infection, and allergies. He reported that the symptoms completely disappeared in 30.3% of the cases, improved significantly in 42.3% of the cases, showed some improvement in 20% of the cases, and showed no signs of improvement in 7.4% of the cases.

In 1966, a hospital in Jerusalem conducted a study involving 38 babies, between the ages of two and twelve months, with about the same degree of respiratory problems. The babies were separated into two groups of nineteen. One group was treated in a room ionised with negative ions, while the second group was handled with the standard treatment, which included drugs and antibiotics. The babies in the group treated with the air purifier generating negative ions were cured of asthma and bronchitis much more quickly than those in the standard treatment group. The babies in the negative ion group were also found to be less prone to rebound attacks. Interesting point observed during treatment of the babies with negative ion-enriched air is that the babies didn't cry as often or as loudly compared to the other group (Soyka, 1991).

Negative ions and Asthma and Synthetics:

Dr. Bernard Watson, professor of medical electronics at Britain's St. Bartholomew's Teaching Hospital in London, said, "Changing the immediate unhealthy ion environment to help asthmatic means changing everything, clothes, sheets, furniture - just everything." He narrated about one of his patients, a girl, aged fourteen at that time, who had begun to suffer from severe migraine because of clothing and then cured it herself.

> "When she grew to adolescence and began to wear, with great pride, nylon bras and panties favoured by most women, she began to suffer from occasional headaches for the first time in her life. When she graduated to slips and night-dresses and pretty nylon blouses, she became a full-fledged migraine sufferer. Her local general practitioner could offer neither explanation nor help beyond suggesting the onset of menstruation as a cause. But the girl was bright enough to associate the clothes of blooming womanhood with her problem and promptly abandoned the feminine underwear and nightdresses. Now her clothes are of cotton, which is the only fibre that creates no charge at all, and of natural fibres like wool, which carry little charge of either kind. However, once migraine has taken root it is not easy to cure" (Watson, 2001)

Christian Bach, an electrical engineer of The Director of the Danish Air Ionization Institute, has studied the clothes and environments of asthmatics and others who suffer from positive ion poisoning, then pinpoints the offending fabrics and articles that are throwing the ion effect out of balance. Bach and his colleagues have worked with many hospitals in treating many victims of asthma and other respiratory ills.

> Bach told a story like that of Dr. Bernard Watson, which has become a classic case history involving a woman who had asthma. Her asthmatic troubles were found in her

own apartment but not of her friends. Even a negative ion generator was of no help. So Bach conducted to find what must be the reason for these odd effects only with a difference of place. The questions arose: Was the culprit the furniture, the television set, the bedding, the lamp shades? Bach found that the lady's taste ran mostly to modern synthetic fabrics. However, that alone was insufficient to explain the problem, so Back began cross-examining the woman about her housekeeping. He found that her furniture was treated with cellulose and silicone-based furniture finishes. Laboratory tests proved that such finishes, when rubbed with polishing rags and dusters, produce a positive charge. Then she visited the friends in whose home her asthma condition disappeared. There she found that the furniture was hand polished with old-fashioned wax and elbow grease, which produced no static charge at all. Bach coated the victim's furniture with an anti-static compound, told her to buy antique furniture without modern wood treatments, and her asthma attacks ceased (Rosalind Tan, 2013).

Bach had an experience in one instance in which he was called in to help a chicken growing farmer. The farmer had two large chicken houses each housing 20,000 chickens. Around 150 and 200 chickens died every week in one of the chicken house. Bach found that both chicken houses were of identical design and construction, except that the one where the chickens died had a roof lined with sheets of plastic while the other had a roof lined of wood. Whenever there was a change in weather the death rate went up. Bach concluded that when the weather changes affected air electricity the plastic stimulated the production of positive ion overdoses. To overcome the positive ions he treated the roof with anti-static substance. Within weeks the chicken mortality rate was normal.

By 1967 Bach had treated almost 1,000 hay fever and asthma cases whose problems were cured or eased by his "passive therapy" approach. In one of the cases a man became an asthma victim because his wife bought two new lampshades that led to overproduction of positive ions. In another instance several members of the same family became sufferers because their new television set had a teak cabinet that had been treated with cellulose, which attracted positive ions.

On Negative ions:

Former NASA scientist James B. Beal, who came across the negative ion problem while studying the type of environment needed in space capsules, wrote: "The human race was developed in ionized air. Nature used the ions in developing our biological processes." In other words, people have been designed to function properly in an environment that contains certain level of ionization.

Removal of dust and germs in agriculture:

Bailey W. Mitchell, an agricultural engineer and veterinarian, Henry D. Stone of Southeast Poultry Research Laboratory under Agricultural Research Service (ARS) are the researchers in Athens, Georgia, USA. They developed the ionizer system in 1994. The developmental project was to find a way to reduce the Salmonella virus and the dust in poultry areas. The method developed was to create a negative ion to mix with the poultry dust of positive ion. This technology might have looked like a common concept but to bring it to action and proving in place was an exciting job. By installing a negative ion generator and passing the air mixed with these charged ions thought the poultry areas, the operation removed the dust. At the same time it reduced the disease producing Salmonella and Newcastle disease virus from the lungs and feathers of the chickens. In the testing, the researchers found the air samples with 95% reduction of Salmonella (Holt, 1999).

Review report on the Negion research:

With all the advantages of negative ions found by so many research groups some are sceptic. One such report by Perez et al is 'Air ions and mood outcomes: a review and meta-analysis'. The report says that 'no consistent influence of positive or negative air ionization over anxiety, mood, relaxation, sleep, and personal comfort measures was observed. Negative air ionization was associated with lower depression scores particularly at the highest exposure level. Future research is needed to evaluate the biological plausibility of this association' (Perez et al, 2013).

Reason for all the doubts or non-acceptance of any sort of negion theory arises due to non-availability of the measuring processes of qualitative parameters. All the mental activities that get improved by the negative ions are of quality oriented and having no measurable quantities. The results of pre and post treatment arrive by observation, opinion, evaluation, inference, assessment and judgment and all are quantitative. Only persons, who are involved with the experiments and who have experience in observation of persons can decide about the results. Any development in the experiment, better or worse, of a non-quantifiable factor from a person or a patient can be recorded with face to face assessments. There can only be a statistical approach in the natural bio-systems.

In such cases of quality judgment, one has to take the primary report as right or wrong or question the researcher to decide right or wrong. Further analysis of the primary reports of the quantified values of the event qualities will lead to low confidence level and the reviews have no values and meaning.

Negions improve the mind and the mind improves the health:

In many ways NEGIONS can improve our health and how we make use of that cosmic energy is up to our intelligence, mentality, capability and ability. What one has to take care always is the HEALTH before onset of the disease than the DISEASE to be treated to recover back one's health.

"The energy of the mind is the essence of life."

-Aristotle-

6

Health and Disease

'Prevention is better than cure'
is the old saying
that is in old books
and has been
forgotten.

Education has improved to a level that
huge money is spent on curing diseases,
but not for preventing them.

More research for medicines,
and new machines to evaluate diseases
but less efforts to promote healthy living.

Many doctors to work with diseases
No doctors to work for health
Many hospitals and no health clinics.

You recognize the value of good health
only when you suffer from disease.

'Prevention is better than cure'

80 *Ko Paandu*

What is Health and What is Disease?

Keeping a thief away is health and searching for a thief with an
identity from a security camera is like seeking a medicine for
a cure from sickness. Building a house with a good protective
doors and windows would not allow a thief into the house.
This is prevention. We build the house weak and then install
good quality cameras to record the traces of the thief. Then
we try to recover the stolen property from the burglar through
the police. This cure after a disease would not result in relief
but unhealthy state. The prevention would have avoided the
creation a thief and the new health problem.

We consider health and disease are the two sides of a coin.
Only with this assumption health is decided. If one has no
disease one is healthy. The modern technology has brought
and continues to develop so many devices to find the diseases.
The time one equipment is developed for a disease many more
diseases are on queue. So far no equipment or instrument has
been developed to certify that a person is healthy. If one does
not have a disease he is considered to be healthy. Based on
this the disease industry is being developed instead of a health
organisation.

How can one be a healthy human being? One can be a
healthy individual without disease taking good food, proven
food, healthy food, herbs and minerals. Also one can take
preventive medicines prior to onset of diseases. In today's life,
the medicines that we consume have grown in proportions
almost like food. The food we consume is shrinking in the
shape of diet, measured and swallowed. Whenever one gets
a disease, the person starts medication and as he gets back
to normal the confidence is a bit shaken. Body and mind
cannot come back to the original state of well-being again.
The individual is prone to anxiety as to when the next disease
might attack him. Peace of mind goes into pieces.

Mind wants to do something but the body may be prevented from action by self or others. Any action that is wanted by the mind be it eating something new, reading, walking, sleeping, buying or even talking, when it gets satisfied there is comfort. Else the difference between the two starts and that lingers in the mind always. Why the mind is important? Mind only wants to do something that fulfils the needs of the body. Body gets the things done through mind. The interest of your mind is not satisfied when your own body is incapable to do something. Also others around you may not co-operate or may dissuade or even stop you in the middle of the activity that you were doing. Basic reason here is the mental agony of not carrying out an action and being denied the expected satisfaction. If you are able to carry out the activity what you thought and the activity is carried out well, there comes the satisfaction. You are at peace.

Whether the reason for the unsatisfactory mind is due to food or any other external matter, the conflict happens between the mind and the actions that were supposed to satisfy you. Same way when something is forced upon you, which you do not want, that force disturbs you. A simple example is, when the basic requirement of milk is forced on a child to drink, the child vomits. When the same child is tempted it demands the same milk or drinks by itself. The child's happiness in drinking makes the acceptance by its body and its digestion smooth.

You eat something that you like most and a few hours later your stomach gives trouble. A disturbance to the mind during eating disturbs the digestion later. Peace and comfort during eating plays a role in digestion. This is a clear disagreement between your mind and your body. Same way forced intake of food creates problems and voluntary eating does not do so. Any disagreement to the mind because of the body, gives rise to an unhealthy condition. What is the uneasiness here? Unhealthy body or unhealthy mind or both are being unhealthy? What is the cause of the disease? What we observe as disease are the symptoms of the basic disease, the result of an unsatisfied mind and the problems that the body faces as its consequence.

Basically a disturbance to the mind or the body is due to some problem in that person. Mind, being the decision maker, attributes any problem to the body as a disease. Mind does not think that it has a disease, when it really has one. A person with a problem of mind has to be understood by another person only. A person with a problem of his body goes to a physician by himself. However, a person who has a problem in his mind thinks that he is perfect and does not feel a need to go to a physician. He has to be taken to a psychiatrist by somebody else.

Our mind-body system has lot of solutions within it to take care of innumerable problems that arise within. At the same time mind gets troubled when body has any flaw. What we say as mind is the conscious one which gets troubled looking for solutions. The background mind, the subconscious, is always working and is taking care of the problems. Our mind-body system fights to clear any problem of the body (BisongGuo, 2002)

As an example, during a walk outside home, one may catch a cold and the cold may be cleared within a few days even without taking any pills. Strong mind cares nothing about the cold and the cold disappears. Weak mind worries and thinks of the cold always and goes to the doctor and it becomes a future disease, next time also trying for the medicine for the same cold. Weak or strong mind is basic and influences further developments in the life. A simple advertisement that draws your attention that you can get well on taking a medicine for flu can make you weak. An advice by a friend not to treat a simple headache and let it get cleared by itself could make you feel strong. A chronic cold every year in winter or summer or when one faces a draft of a wind is not what we describe here. An acute problem becomes a disease when there is worry in the mind; else, it disappears as the common cold. In many cases simple symptoms are amplified and brought to the category of big disease. Chronic cold has many causes including the basics of the body of an individual and bad treatment of the acute cold in the past. The mind only decides whether the cold is a disease or a simple discomfort that disappears the next day.

A problem which our body continues fighting is the chronic problem. If we notice the problem as an issue for us, it is a disease. There are many problems existing in the body which we do not know and do not notice. We detect the problem only when our senses are able to observe and perceive that there is disturbance. Also diseases are found when one goes to the doctor for some problem. The doctor is able to watch some major issue in that person. This may be due to the observation of the experienced physician or the observation of the laboratory results, what the machines and laboratory tests on your body fluids reveal. Many people, by taking medicines for simple troubles of the body create problems for themselves as the medicines taken in by them result later on in a chronic problem.

From an observation to a prescription:

The present day treatment of a patient by our medical system goes as follows. An individual come to a decision that he has some difficulty and may think and name that as a disease. The person makes a visit to a physician. Patient tells his symptoms, observations and the feelings, the three important indicators of the unhealthy condition of an individual. The doctor is focused on the values and quantities of the condition of the body rather than the qualitative observations as narrated by the person. Physician wants tests of body products, blood, stool, urine etc., and inner parts by x-rays and scans as the results of what the machines can watch. The lab tests fix the values in numbers with what is normal, minimum required and the maximum not to exceed and the machines give the measurements of sizes of the body parts. What would be more appropriate to be considered by physician here would be the cause of the problems based on the description of symptoms by the patient and the test results. But the tabulated and recorded results from the laboratory tell how the body chemistry is and the physiology stands as at that time of the test. The results of tests and opinions of specialists make the physician to conclude a name for the disease rather than base his decision also on the mind of the patient. A disease once concluded automatically decides the medicines in line with the experience of the doctor.

What would be a better way to treat the patient? The physician is supposed to observe the symptoms of the patients. Some can be observed physically and some cannot. Observations made by the patient on his own body or how is his feeling should also be considered by the doctor. Some observations might have existed before the visit to the clinic and noticed by the patient and that may not exist now. Often times, the patient's narrative of problems may or may not be clear in his observations and symptoms and has to be deduced by the doctor after further questioning. Few doctors correlate all this information along with the observations made on the body like pain, itching, giddiness etc. while drawing his conclusion. The test results are from the body and the narrations are from the mind. Many depend only on the lab results. More importance is given for the quantified lab records than the symptoms and narrations and disease is decided. Most of the diseases are named following from the symptoms and may not be the root cause. Finally the prescription is based on the lab test values. The medicines are supposed to bring the next lab results post treatment to normal. With such expectations, the prescription is finally written by the doctor.

Some persons are healthy and some face lot of health issues even though they live in the same locality, exposed to same environment or even within same house. Each person of the same family gets into different health problems. Some live long and some live short. Any health problem is connected with that person's mind and body. Nowadays, as per the present medicine system, body is the one causing disease due to bacteria and virus and so that body is the one to be treated. In reality however, mind being the controller and is the deciding authority, mind should also be considered while treating the body and an improvement in overall health will take care automatically.

Sources of Diseases.... Where from one gets all these diseases? They are like past, present and future and are the Hereditary, Acquired and Manmade.

Hereditary disease cannot be avoided. We observe many diseases in us that our parents or grandparents had. Proving by somebody by theory and experimentation goes strong in our mind. Gregor Mendel, in 1865, published his observations on hybridization of pea plants. He developed the principles describing the characters that were transferred to the next generation by colour and shape of peas. By this way Mendel laid the foundation for heredity. His theory is consistent with inherited human diseases. In 1900 by Carl Correns, Hugo de Vries and Erich Tschermak, demonstrated that the heritage is transferred from parent to their issues.

In 1902 Walter Sutton and Theodor Boveri had independently outlined the chromosomal theory. British physician, Archibald Garrod, published his observations on the disease, alkaptonuria. He established a link deducing that alkaptonuria was inherited from the families he studied. In 1911 E.B.Wilson mapped the colour blindness gene to the X-chromosome. We gained the knowledge from a very basic understanding of the rules of heredity and genes to the completed sequence of the human genome, the ultimate gene map, within a period of ten decades. Later chromosomes and DNA (DeoxyriboNucleic Acid) came into the picture to prove those theories. Chromosomes are complex structures that have the DNA in an orderly and consistent arrangement within the nucleus of the cell (Bateson, 1902).

Major force acting in a person is based on his heredity. Every human being is unique. That is the reason every individual is different from the other even if born at the same time, same place and even as twins. Nature automatically produces everything as a unique product. Even flowers from a tree are different. One flower may look like the other but differs in size, petals, and layers and in so many ways. Take apples from the same tree or same branch or stem or twig. No two apples will be exactly same. This is the way human beings are made by nature. We are unique products and can be differentiated in so many ways. One way we ourselves are differentiating is finger prints at present. In contrast whatever man produces are from moulds and industrial products. It may be very costly for us to make the products unique.

Every individual has his own constitution such as mental makeup, body structure and the hidden health. The health and diseases of the forefathers may have impact over the person. Predominantly the hereditary nature plays an important part in acquired diseases.

Acquired diseases can be avoided by better food and health practices. They are caused by neighbours, from epidemics, one's intolerance from environment like rain, sun etc. Diseases created by environment and epidemics etc. can be managed but not always. Not everybody in a place gets affected by epidemics. Hence the basic nature of a person has a lot of role in acquired diseases too. Even the bad habits of an individual have the base from heredity, the root. You are driving the car in a good road and do regular maintenance. The car runs well. The same vehicle parked in sun and rain without proper shelter and when driven by you in dirty roads with muddy water, gets involved in accidents due to your bad driving. Then the car shows problems and it is created by you as if acquired from environment. This is same as the diseases that are acquired from outside based on the way you live, for which the basic reason is your life style and attitude. Apart from the heredity deciding the basic character of a person it is one of the important factors in the acquired diseases (Kennedy, 2001).

Manmade diseases are diseases knowingly or unknowingly caused by others and side effects of medicines. Side effects may or may not be known to the physician or to drug manufacturers. Many new diseases are out of the manmade medicines. Also bad treatment by the medical system and taking wrong medicines etc. also creates diseases subsequently. Even with your perfect driving skills somebody on the road makes a rash accident with your car and that is manmade problem, like you are party to an accident caused by others without your knowledge. This is manmade and not your heredity or acquired.

One who eats any food that he is used to, no craving or rejection occurs and food gets digested and will have no problems. When mind and body disagree, degradation of health sets in. You like something and you eat. Just see the event. Mind likes. Body is supposed to digest. If it helps to do, the health goes fine. Why mind likes something? Mind likes because body needs something from that food due to the experience it had in previous consumptions. If the body cannot digest it may create some problem such as stomach pain, headache, ulceration etc. This is a direct case of violation or disagreement with the mind. It indicates that a deficiency or disease exists already. Not that a disease is created. Just that it is announced now. Existing deficiency will appear only when the mind and body together cannot solve. Mind and body work together a lot for so much time and only when they get fed up, mind feels that as a problem and announced. Now some external action needs to be taken, namely seek some treatment.

Let us take a look how mind and body tries to resolve the problem of deficiency. Body wants so many minerals, many compounds with vitamins, starch for energy, air to breathe, ions for energized activities, good environment etc. The mind requests and the body takes in and digests and in that process converts the materials from various foods to the forms required for the body. In this process so many mechanisms are involved. The minerals are absorbed and converted to various forms of salts, as required in the body system. Say calcium from one form of salt or from a mineral is converted to calcium phosphate, calcium carbonate and the same way sodium compounds are transformed to chloride, phosphate and sulphate of sodium etc. Also minerals like iron, zinc, selenium etc. takes various forms of salts and goes as part of other molecules. The metals in the body are in some form of salt and not as metal. Many are part of vitamins and other compounds. Metal particles enter in our body in unnatural way from wastes of industries and they create lot of health issues. To get the various salts in its required form to the cells of the body, the mechanism connected with that conversion shall be working and shall have better efficiency to receive a required amount.

In 1880s, Dr. Wilhelm Heinrich Schuessler, a German doctor, believed that a deficiency in one or more of twelve salts led to the disease in the body. He discovered that the health of the cells in the body depends on a particular amount of twelve inorganic salts (iron phosphate, sodium chloride, calcium fluoride, silica etc) in them. Any deficiency or differences from the normal amount of these inorganic salts lead to the unhealthy state (Schuessler, 1914).

Let me explain with an example of a human made machine in comparison with our nature made body. Our body is similar to any other engine of a motor vehicle. Like we eat and walk, the automobile engines eat fuel and rolls on the road. Both have lots of similarities. Engine is invented by man and so he can rectify and there is specialist for each type of engine. All engines of one model vehicle are alike and repairing is easy by few trained persons. We, as Humans are unique and every individual is a different type of human engine. We have to repair ourselves and hence we have doctors as specialists. For a car engine to work so many supports are required apart from fuel. Fuel has to burn to impart force to the gear-train and to the wheels finally. Fuel has to be injected to the engine from fuel tank and spark ignition continuously to burn the fuel. The engine's rotation has to be transmitted to the wheels through the gears. The heat of engine and gears are to be removed by coolants. Tires shall be cool and with good grips to the road. Our body mechanism is also like that of the vehicle engine, food as the fuel and energy transmitted to the muscles in our legs, hands and so many parts finally. In between there exists many mechanisms which works 24 hours even when we stay in one place. Vehicle engine is inorganic and in comparison our body is an organic mechanism.

You face a problem with your car after about a year and take it to a garage. The serviceman tells you that this is due to a manufacturing defect and the car managed it so far even though the defect existed. The garage mechanic says "a bad welding is found now and it has broken now. That is from a factory fabrication shop. Now we have to weld and cannot say if it can have the quality like the original from the manufacturing floor of the factory." Also the garage engineering manager says "If you go to the Factory qualified shop in the city the repair would be done removing the factory deficiency". This is like the individual's hereditary problem and like this many others may be in the car and we may not notice until the car shows a drag in its running. We, the individuals may have many such problems from the factory of nature that we may not notice.

Assume the engine is perfect and all mechanisms of fuel injection, gears, cooling system and tires are 100 % (percent) efficient. You need the minimum fuel to drive. You can run it for Miles and kilometres. Same way you eat minimum food and you are healthy.

If the machine has an engine problem or never reaches the expected speed can we inject more fuel? Yes. Sometimes we do if tire pressure is low and dragging or gear is having more friction or coolant is not removing the heat. More fuel will push the engine to the required speed. Our human body is also running like this sometimes with reduced efficiencies. But beyond certain limit fuel or food cannot work.

Before going to the physician, let me explain the efficiency of the mechanism a bit more in detail with an example of one of the constituent of the mineral. Our body does not take metals directly. Body needs the natural product in the form of metallic salts. One of the metallic salts known as table salt is the basic need for your body. The salt is part of the food and your mind knows about it based on the taste you had some time before. You crave for the specific food that contains the salt, you need. Sometime back you were eating the same food in a normal way. The body by taking the food before knows that that specific food has the required metallic salt which will get converted to the required ingredient. Now you need more of that salt. More than the normal as if that is the food you require more than others. Any amount of eating never stops the craving. But the body digests well. It shows there is problem in the body that wants something from that food. Hence the mind craves. There is no disease as the problem is not appearing to you. You are finally fed up of eating the same food and stop one day. Some people will continue to eat more of the same food. Why?

Love - Hate attitudes:

What is love and what is hate and why it happens in same place? The one you would hate most is the one you loved most at some stage of your life. Your mind and body are in love to have liking for food and digestion for energy. If a warm, affectionate love and bonding as friendship exists all through the life, the mind and body would get along well.

Many people who love to eat eggs in their youth or drink more milk in childhood would

> **Love and Hate:**
>
> A boy likes a girl. Love blossoms between them. Everything is fine until one day due to some problem there is negligence on the part of the girl. Attitude of the boy changes now. Boy starts to show more interest towards the girl and more attachment else the girl might go away. The girl somehow does not get on well with the boy. With all his efforts the boy could not win and suddenly he hates the girl. Why? This is the love hate attitude also seen in nature.

stop later in life abruptly. Also one who never took eggs or drank milk or ate meat will start imbibing them at later age. This is same as food craving explained before. The craving or rejection is talked here and not the normal food intakes. The theory here is connected with the efficiency of the mechanism that converts the food to get required ingredient. The mechanism has less efficiency and so needs more intakes. One can notice many persons would eat less and would carry many activities and also healthy. In case the ingredient derived is sufficient, the mechanism would continue to work with its efficiency. The person would continue to eat the food in the same way. The time the efficiency of the mechanism deteriorates more intake of the substance would be required. Only then the required output to the body system would be available. On any decrease in efficiency would increase the work of the conversion mechanism. At some stage the body mechanism would get tired and gives up. That indicates inefficiency of the mechanism, which went bad due to overwork or bad inputs or no energy to work etc.

What is efficiency? If a car is designed with an engine to run 16 kilometres (10 miles) with one litre of fuel with all its parts working well as designed, means 100% (percent) efficient. If the mileage gets reduced to 8 kilometres the efficiency is 50%. To get the same mileage of 16 km car needs 2 litres now. More intake to meet the needs and there is a limit for fuel injection to ensure complete combustion. The values in examples given here are for easy understanding. Example of overall car efficiency is applicable to individual's body mechanisms. Our body has lot of individual mechanisms. Even with more fuel the car cannot run to that value expected and has to be sent for servicing.

Assume the mechanism that converts the food to the required ingredient is getting bad and the efficiency is thus reduced. To compensate the need one has to take in more of that specific food. Conversion capacity may get reduced slowly by decreased efficiency and the mechanism finds it difficult to function and gets fed up due to being overworked. The human system has to feed energy for all the mechanisms of the body and the specific mechanism in this example is tired even though not stopped working but needs repair by the physician. This is akin to a fuel filter getting clogged. Filter is not working and so less fuel and car is not running, but the filter can be cleaned.

Let us see the conversion mechanism example by using values for some better understanding. Example taken here is magnesium intake even though magnesium required for body is in different forms, magnesium phosphate, magnesium sulphate etc.

One adult may need magnesium and takes almonds to meet the requirement. As long the mechanism that converts the almonds to required magnesium salt everything goes fine. When mechanism has problem and efficiency is reduced. Intakes of almond would increase. At one stage mechanism gets tired. Person cannot consume that much almond and the mechanism also would find it difficult to work and assimilate. The foods get rejected, namely the almonds. Mind will try some other source of magnesium and that mechanism may be different. Also the efficiency will be different for each food that contains magnesium, cashew nut, Almonds, peanut, banana etc. If conversion efficiency is increased and magnesium absorbed is more, then there will be a reduction in intake of magnesium contained food. With this we can find the reason that children will be able consume any new food item with interest resulting in good digestion and not old people.

> **Magnesium from Almonds:**
> One adult may need around 420 mg (one gram equals to 1000 mg, milligrams) of magnesium. Assume this person in example takes only almonds for required magnesium of the body. The person eats 350 grams of almonds with each gram of the nut containing nearly 3 mg of magnesium with a total of around 1050 mg for 350 grams of the nut. The person in this example is assumed to have the body mechanism with efficiency of 40%. Hence out of 1050 mg of magnesium in the nut consumed, 420 mg (approx.) is absorbed in the body. This is fine for an average man. When the conversion efficiency is decreased to 20% one has to consume 700 g almonds. If still worse, consumption will be 1Kg if the efficiency goes down to 15%. Person cannot consume that much and the mechanism also would find it difficult to work.
>
> Need is 420 mg per day. 3 mg from 1 gram of Almond. 1050 mg from 350 g of Almond. In conversion efficiency is only 40%. Body gets 1050 x (40/100)= 420 mg. If efficiency is 20% you need 2x350 g ie. 700 g of almond

The deficiency of mechanism of magnesium by reduced efficiency creates a triggering in the mind or craving to consume more of the food with magnesium. More food is more work for the mechanism and machine gets tired. Feedback from body is to reject the food. Now the person is devoid of magnesium. Hence the person may become magnesium deficient. Else the mind will search to consume some other magnesium content food elsewhere. This example of interest and rejection can be seen in salt eating persons. One who was eating more salt, milk, yogurt etc. would hate to consume the salt, milk, yogurt etc. at some stage in life.

Many times the mind and the attitude of the kids could find new foods and also consume easily and the system will adjust for absorbing magnesium. This would help the kid at later stage of life to adapt to different type of foods. Specific food at younger age would make adapting any new food at old age difficult or impossible. In old aged persons there is no force and drive to find a new food with magnesium content. Young age is the one which forms mechanisms and tuned for later life. That is the reason kids should be tempted to taste and eat any type of eatables mainly vegetables, fruits and nuts so that they are ready with many type of mechanisms developed in the body. The persons who have practiced to eat variety of food at younger age will have in their memory to find alternative resources for the requirement in the food at old age. This is similar to the resistance a body prepares itself to fight a disease at any stage with inoculation at an early age.

Allergy is a simple mechanism here. By eating something one gets a problem, reason being the bad mechanism of conversion. We think that specific food is the allergen. The food which creates allergy is the food one requires. The allergy problem happens only when the required contents of food consumed is not converted properly. The time the conversion mechanism fails there is no way the body can utilise the food. When this food becomes extra burden for the body reaction is in two ways. One is no liking for food and no interest even to eat. Another action is the body continuously tries to resolve. In trying so many other mechanisms work hard and failure happens. This requires the resolution of conversion mechanisms. Basically the food that is allergic has some important content in it required by the person.

The disease is like an enemy. Allergy is like an enemy. To resolve the issue with the enemy is to deal with that rival some way or other and clear the issue. Resolving is the solution and pending to resolve or avoiding or rejecting the enemy is like retaining the disease. Unresolved issue will make you remember the enemy always.

Disease basket:

The diseases are seen as symptoms and each symptom or group of symptoms are named as a disease. Medicines are prescribed for a person's symptoms without finding the specific mechanism for rectification. Doctors may advice to take more magnesium (example) contained food. But this may cripple the mechanism and new symptom would appear that may lead to new disease. Real need is to repair the defective mechanism.

Disease is like a waste basket with first dirt in and the last dirt out. Disease accumulated in our body is First in - Last out type. This is like a waste basket. Five days waste in a basket will be down in the layers with today's waste at the top. Five day old dirt would be at the bottom most. Yesterday's waste would be hiding below the today's waste. Disease stays in our body when not treated well and another disease stays over it hiding the old. Old disease was suppressed because of the incorrect medicine consumed, else would have disappeared. When any disease is suppressed instead of cure disease becomes part of waste basket. By this way many diseases accumulate one above the other. The last disease appears in front at any time and that is the one that would make us fall in sickness.

Many skin problems that were a common occurrence years back is now no more prevalent. Nowadays babies are born without skin problems. How come old generations had these skin diseases and present day boys and girls are free from them. Parents had them but their children do not have now. Where did it go? Nowhere! Some medicines taken by the parents hid them and some of their children also would be hiding them as their diseases are hereditary.

We are conditioned mentally to believe that Health is to get relieved from a disease of the body. It is true, if we are treated and cured of the disease. Even without any disease when one is mentally upset what happens. Is it a disease? This is not. But the mental worry drives the body to a bad state inviting some problem. Mind is the root cause of many health problems

Disease layers:

Disease has its own layers in appearance from childhood to adulthood. Any individual will have the next problem in a particular pattern based on his weakness of his body mechanisms. Disease is like a leak in the water line due to some problem in the water system. Water always leaks in first weakest part. When the first leak is plugged next weakest part starts to leak and is usually interpreted as it is another problem or another disease. It is very much apparent that the underlying reason is same. Next leak is another problem and another disease and so on. Without finding the reason for the water leak we start plugging the lines and the leak continues in another next weakest part. The time the first hole is plugged the reason for the high pressure in the water line should also be found. Normally this is not done. Reason may be that the pump itself is running faster, there may be a block in pipeline downstream or a bad valve that opened more water into the pipe. If the pump is running at high speed and pressurizing the line, then that has to be attended. Else by the time we are plugging the hole in the pipe line, pump may stop or could get damaged. When the symptoms are treated to make them disappear the root-cause is forgotten.

Instead of searching the cause and resolving, we work on the symptoms, naming them as new diseases and clearing them from our vision and hiding them. At one time most of the individuals would have only one disease and many symptoms. Like one disease basket contains many types of dirty items.

If we examine the history of the diseases of the population, problems that started from simple skin eruptions gravitate slowly towards kidney failure, the last important drain line mechanism of the body. Lot of developments had taken place after the heart transplants in recent times. The skin problem is at the bottom of the disease basket and basket is growing big and large with more diseases piling up.

A sample disease and its theory:

An example of a disease will help to understand the root and its symptoms. As a major problem in the life of the people, asthma is one of the diseases. Let us see the probable root cause of an asthmatic person. Asthmatic patients are told that allergens and irritants are the problem. If asthma is a disease, reason for that shall be one root cause. Patients are told that Asthma symptoms can be prevented by avoiding indoor allergens such as dust mites, cockroaches, animal dander, and mould (a fungus), pollens from trees, grasses, and flowers, irritants such as cigarette smoke, air pollution, low air quality from factors such as traffic pollution, high ozone levels, cat fur, synthetic fibres, chemicals or dust in the workplace, compounds in home decor products, sprays (such as hairspray) and more. Major problem in the house are the transparent and hidden from the eyes are the house dust mites which are 0.3 mm only long due to glued carpets, heat and insulations (WDDTY-Asthma manual).

What is common here is what all symptoms lead to for the person, difficulty in breathing. All the above allergens and irritants are making the atmosphere around the person devoid of something in air, likely the negions. Asthma patients cannot tolerate this and suffer to breathe.

One can notice well that Asthma patients are very sensitive and will get triggered by even small events and simple talks. Basically it is mind connected. To have good energy for the mind more negative ions are needed for an asthmatic. The allergens, which are positively charged particles absorb the negative ions and get neutralized. Now the surrounding has less negions because of all ion absorbing materials. To have more negions, asthmatic person needs more air because of less efficiency in converting the negative ions in air to the use inside the body. However any individual's capacity to breathe is limited. More air is not possible to be breathed in by one to take more ions. The person needs more negatively ionized particles in the air that the person breathes.

There is one temporary solution for an asthmatic patient and that is a negative ion generator. The permanent cure is to find the bad mechanism and rectify. The mechanism for each individual may be different and hence the medicine would be different from individual to individual.

Without understanding whether we have a disease or not we take pills, capsules and injections just for a simple symptom of pain, tiredness, headache, fever, cold or cough. These medicines escalate the problem or suppress or hide the existing problem and create new problems to be termed as another disease or diseases.

Modern life started using chemical as a major resource for the comforts in homes, residences, transports, toys, furniture and mainly in food. The same chemicals once thought giving comfort, started showing their true colors after a gap of few years, by which time, health has started its degradation depositing the chemicals in the body and affecting us for a long time. New chemicals are coming up with assurances such as proven, tested in approved labs, certified by government agencies, best for human health and are human friendly. The mess created out of this are known only after few years when they show their ugly head in front of the gloomy human face by which time it is probably too late for any remedy.

Famous chemical in Kitchen utensil and in Food –PFOA:

One of the famous TEFLON coated utensils of the yester years had wide spread use. It had the ability due to its non-sticking character to catch the attention of the people to find a place as part of the utensil stand in every kitchen. Only those who could not afford these utensils and those who lived in remote corners of the earth untouched by development are still unable to see the uses of TEFLON coated products. The people in remote areas may still be using the mud pots for cooking.

Recent research has found links between PFOA (PerFluoroOctanoic Acid), a chemical in TEFLON of Dupont Company and female infertility, low sperm count, high cholesterol and a cause for thyroid problems. The thyroid gland is like your body's control centre, regulating everything from heart rate to body temperature and supporting reproduction, mental health, digestion, and metabolism. So deep is the health impact by use of this thirty year old product as is revealed now.

US EPA (Environmental Protection Agency) has listed the PFOA as a likely carcinogen. With all these findings, no current restrictions exist on the use of PFOA in consumer products. The chemical is used to repel heat, water, grease, and stains, and is used extensively in cookware and in flame-resistant and waterproof clothing. PFOA is used also in

- Greasy fast-food wrappers, one of people's greatest exposure to PFOA
- Egg breakfast sandwiches boasted the highest levels.
- Pizza boxes have also been shown to have a chemical non-stick coating.

- Hardwood floors over carpeting coated with stain-repelling chemicals.
- Microwave-popcorn bags are often coated with non-stick chemicals.
  (LEAH ZERBE, 2013)

What are the causes for the diseases? Theory is that virus and bacteria are the causes of diseases. The research in disease and medicine has gone too far and the theory remains untouched. A person having a problem with his body or mind has an illness but normally unhealthy condition of a person's body is called an illness. The problems of an individual are categorised as Disease, Illness, Disorder, Syndrome etc. All the problems of a sick person are connected to that individual and shall be put in group and a cure shall be found. That is however not the case in treatments given in recent times. The mental conditions such as tiredness, depression, sleepiness, drowsiness, fatigue, exhaustion, inattentiveness are not considered important by the physician. These are not linked with the problems of body in deciding the prescription of medicines. The resolution of the doctor is that the body problems cause mental ill health.

Always the search for a bacteria or virus is prime importance in the lab tests. Some health issues connected with the body arises due to mental issues. But the treatment is only for the body. 'Does a bacterium cause the disease or disease causes the bacteria' is a question raised by many. A child when it gets afraid of something gets a fever. Even adults get fever or shivering when they are afraid of some grave danger. But the routine followed in treating is the search for bacteria or virus.

Day by day more diseases come to the list due to so many reasons. If the disease basket is not cleaned, then and there, basket would become full and overflow and the basket itself would get destroyed and buried eventually.

If health has to be improved and disease has to be avoided, primary concern shall be with the individuals' heredity. The weakest and strongest parts of the body are the part of the person's structure and build up from his birth. This is embedded in the body constitution of an individual. Care shall be taken in ensuring proper diet and healthy habits in individuals from child hood so as to prevent disease and start finding and clearing the disease basket to reduce the height of the dirt, than let it pile up. Then healthy individuals can roam around this earth in their healthy bodies with radiant and glowing faces.

We have gained more knowledge on diseases than the wisdom to avoid ill health. Our body and its constitution are as we inherited from our forefathers. We inherited good health at birth as our forefathers used to eat healthy and lived healthy free from diseases. Unless we gain knowledge of what we humans were using as our energy source for long, changing our food to new fast technological stuff would downgrade ourselves in health. We should not forget that the major energy is from good, natural, organic, pesticide less, herbicide less, chemical less FOOD.

Before you tell the truth to the patient,
be sure you know the truth
And the patient wants to hear it

-Chinese proverb-

7

Food

The earth can exist without
minerals, plants, animals and human race.

Minerals can exist without plant, animals and human beings
Plants can exist without animals and human population
Animals can live without humans.

But
human race cannot live without
Minerals,
Plants
or
Animals.

Source of Food
as
energy for humans is
derived only from the
Earth,
Minerals, Plants and Animals.

Food for a traveller going on a pilgrimage:

During the days of yore, for many centuries when kings ruled India in small kingdoms, pilgrims, saints, and common folk used to go by walk for several days to visit the sacred places of worship or to visit their own relatives. Only the rich could afford horses and chariots for their travels. Walking was the most common mode of travel for the common folks to move from place to place and to reach their destination. The

> **Rudraksha maala:**
>
> A garland made from the seeds of a tree whose Botanical name is Elaeocarpus ganitrus.
>
> This tree is grown in Nepal, Thailand, Burma and Indonesia. This has characteristic of having a magnetic field and can be tested easily. Keep a copper coin on a wooden table and keep the Rudraksha over the coin. Bring a second coin from above and close to the seed. The seed will give a small twist.

travel used to take from few days to even few months to reach the destination. Kings felt that it was their duty or dharma for the upkeep of such sacred places of worship and to assist the pilgrims, they had built resting houses called *'choultry'* (also called Chatram, chaawadi, chowry depending on the region) to provide shelter and food. Some charitable organisations also arranged shelters on the road side. After an overnight stay, pilgrims would continue their journey on foot. In localities where resting houses were not available, the travellers would seek food or shelter from local villagers. How the traveller would ensure that the food, they receive from total strangers is suitable to them? The saints knew a method to judge whether the food would be safe for consumption.

Keeping the food in front, on a leaf (banana leaf, assembled frm leafs of banyan tree), the saint would hold a 'R*udrakshamaala*' above the food and do a prayer. He would hold the garland in his right hand and hang it right over the food, with his eyes half-closed and see the action of the garland. If it rotates clockwise the food was accepted from the host and then would follow a good rest for the night. This activity was done in ever so subtle manner that its significance was known only to a few with no offence meant to the host who served the meal.

The food is categorised as having good energy, bad energy and neutral or null. Poisoned foods, decayed foods with fungus are considered negative foods with bad energy and a bad smell will emanate and the *Rudrakshamaala* would rotate anti-clockwise. This includes food containing Garlic and Onion too. Even though garlic and onion are used as herbs for healing they are considered as bad in the daily intake by some pious people. Chillies belong to the null category. Other food is considered good and fit for the stomach and is the positive food.

As you sow, so shall you reap:

Characteristics of the food from a plant has the character of the plant from which it is produced, may be a leaf, raw vegetable, fruit, nut or another part of plant. One who eats that food has that character. Hence a person is built of many characters from mineral to animals. The plants or animals have life energy in them and the same energy comes to our body. The chemicals have null energy. We may think that things occurring in nature on the surface of the earth are inanimate and have no life. Even a stone in its natural form has energy. The common salt sodium chloride has bio energy, but not the elements sodium or chlorine, which have only chemical energy.

Our understanding of the creation in nature and our knowledge of how to use them is rather limited. Let us ponder on the following for a while. A bird builds a nest. Who taught that skill to that bird, the design, the structure, where to build, what materials to be used etc? Is there any source for that bird to learn? Does the bird receive any teaching from other birds? In case of sickness what do they do? If a dog is sick it stops the food. Sometimes it eats grass or the leaves of some plants. How does the dog know? How do the plants take their food? Do they take in and absorb whatever that exists in the soil? What knowledge it has to select specific minerals and salts to lift from the earth and water to the leaves and fruits. Animals teach their calves only for a short time and leave them free. But humans are taught for years. How bees make honey and ants collect their foods perfectly? Animals and plants sense the humidity, rain and earth tremors in advance. They know what food to take from the earth and plants. Some carnivorous animals would not eat another carnivorous animal. The insects live and survive even when we are destroying them. The stones and minerals live long. We think they are lifeless and useless. But they feed energy to us as metallic salts. The much boasted sixth sense in human being is used in analysis, learning and advancement of knowledge, whereas the birds, animals and plants do not learn anything from us. They have natural instincts that are ingrained and maintained in them for generations. We have learnt more in the field of science and technology. With our advanced product, the pesticide, we kill the pests and insects, but the insects have learnt how to survive and to propagate their generations for such a long time.

We, as humans, also have lived for past several generations guided by our natural instincts and our understanding of nature based on observations. The recent advancement of scientific knowledge has eroded all that nature's wealth inherited by us over generations. We lost the natural instincts once we gained knowledge on the nature through science and we turned a blind eye to our instincts. Food selection used to be based on smell, look, colour, size and feel, what we comprehend through our senses. A good food has good smell and bad foods like decayed foods smell foul. This sense of smell has been lost now. What food should be eaten is also influenced by somebody. We are advised what to eat, what not to eat. We are even forced to eat at times by others. Who is intelligent? We think we are - Are we really? Why then are we feeling so much swayed by others? We have to regain the old natural sense that helped us to discriminate what to eat and what to abstain from and only then would we have an energetic mind and a healthy body.

Energy from Food:

Food is the fuel supply to the body to energize all the cells of the body. Food alone cannot make the energy for the body. Each cell is a small engine where fuel is burnt with the oxygen, carried by the blood from lungs and heart. The energized cells keep the body live and active. During this process, characteristic of the cell also changes, based on the type of food. These characters along with the deficiencies in the body are what are passed on to the next generation as heredity. Our heredity by this way is passed to the coming generation.

During this process of energy conversion, many minerals from its natural form gets assimilated into the cells as required. Body needs so many salts and compounds and human instinctive nature is to search and find them to survive. Until the development of science we were eating the food without knowing what it contains, how food digests, how body works etc. Now we know something because of the developments in science. The research in food started finding what the contents are, what is their purpose, how that affects our health etc.

Ingredients of food:

Research has found
- Calories for various foods.
- Vitamins A, B,(B1,B2,B3, B5, B6, B7, B9, B12) C, D, E, K. Some vitamins were renamed also like Vitamin G (Ribofalvin) is now vitamin B2.

- Minerals such as boron, calcium, chromium, cobalt, copper, iodine, iron, magnesium, manganese, molybdenum, nickel, phosphorus, potassium, selenium, silicon, sodium, sulphur, zinc etc. All minerals will be in their natural form occurring as salts. For example sodium occurs as Sodium chloride.
- Some minerals like chromium, copper, iodine, iron, selenium, and zinc are called trace minerals, but essential for human body.
- Cholesterols - LDL and HDL
- Special components such as beta-carotene, Omega-3 fatty acids etc.
- Importance of water for human body even if its Calorie value is zero

Before knowing about the vitamins, minerals, Omega-3 etc., we were consuming food and living for millennia. Research progressed fast during the last few decades on food and medicines for improvement in heath sector –like identification of Vitamin A (Retinol- Cod liver oil) was discovered in 1913 and Vitamin B7 (in Folic acid) in 1941 and so on. Future research may add more and more, as with time our scientific instruments are able to penetrate and measure deep inside the food chain. All the vitamins and minerals are interrelated and more research may lead to revelations of more vitamins and metallic salts in future.

Source of Food:

What we eat as food used to be harvested from the fields and used to reach our kitchen. Now it is being routed as food from the supermarkets. We may not know how our forefathers found the food and the plants that produce edible food grains, fruits, nuts, vegetables etc. That was when science did not exist in the present format. With our present development in technology, the number of new edible items we have found may be zero compared to those established by older generation as food plants and its products. Hence the improvement started in using the existing food. Food industry developed methods to store them for long periods of time. The research found about 40 nutrients and many may get added in future. When fat is still in controversy, the research found that vegetable fat, either saturated or unsaturated, is good and that is the reason the vegetarians, who do not eat meat are less prone to heart problems. The cholesterol is linked to the balance of Low density (LDL) and High density (HDL) Lipoproteins and the research is going deep to find more and to find what they do in our body. Main research in food is to use the existing food products with additions and subtractions of minerals, colors, preservatives etc. Apart from this research goes in attractive packing, playthings for kids as attachments, cute advertisements that should attract attention in the super markets etc. The industry started making packed ready-to-eat foods for all from the babies to adults. Adding to the business advantage, the health issues made the industry to develop foods with importance of vitamins and minerals. Food supplements are its results. The attraction of foods with energy labels as packaged foods has reached the people easily with the help of the media. Even vegetables started to be sold in packets as cut-vegetables and cooked foods with ready to eat labels (Encyclopedia of food).

What does the food research do now is not finding new plants that delivers edible food but to analyse the existing food items deep to the cell, molecule and atom level to find what it is. The additions with food are the preservatives, colours and other chemicals that help us to store for a long time and to make colouring, shape etc. to make it visually more appetising. The ultimate goal the science and the industries have is to exercise the control over food. Then to decide what the public should eat? In the family level, choice of the food and what and when to feed the children was decided by parents. Nowadays, that selection is made by children themselves due to all pervasive media and the television advertisements and mothers lost their control. Later in life, the control over the food is taken over by the doctors and dieticians. Finally, it is by the marketing wings of food companies that tell you what is supposedly good for you, while knowing deep within themselves that it is only meant to boost their business profit margins. As per 1997 survey by National Centre for Health Statistics, US, the diet plays an important part in the deaths by Heart disease, Cancer, Stroke and Diabetes which stand among the top 10 diseases (Rizza, Robert, 2002).

What to eat:

Eating variety of natural produce is the best for health. Individuals eat the food based on the habit from childhood learned from parents and the surrounding society where they were raised. The food consumed by the community is developed based on the availability around the locality and prevalent weather conditions. The easy way of transport added more food items from far-flung regions.

> **Calorie:**
>
> One Food calorie is one kcal (kilo calorie) and is about 1.163×10^{-3} KWh.
> 1KWh means 1 unit of energy.
> 1 unit = 859 kcal.
>
> 1 Unit of energy (normally counted in electrical meters in houses to calculate power consumption) is equivalent to a energy consumed by 100 watts lamp in 10 hours.

When medical industry started giving importance to food, the analysis of food started to find details and contents of every food item. The energy a food can supply to the body in digestion is the main criteria for health.

Food values in Calorie:

Understanding the energy in the food would help the people who measure, weigh and eat. The unit of energy is Calorie. One calorie in food packet label is one food calorie, also called large calorie and is exactly one Kilo calorie (1000 calorie). This is long time confusion and some food packets nowadays label them with kcal. The theory on calculation of calories is changing and the value it represents is only an approximate energy. Patients are told that they need a specific amount of calorie and dieticians are the advisers.

Dieticians advise the patients to eat specific food items. These specifics are based on the persons' health after calculating the calories of each food. Same way some individuals are advised for weight reduction. An average person needs an intake of food with 2000 to 2500 Kilo calories. Not all the food would be converted to energy, but with all the efficiency with a person one needs about 20% of the energy for the brain activity. Brain is the major consumer of energy.

The significance a calorie has in our food would give an idea about what we eat and drink. To start with an important food item, water, plain water, has zero calories. Only the small amount of salt in water which gives the taste has some calories. Even with no calorie, water is a must for our body system.

At present, the method used is called Atwater system to find the amount of calorie in food by finding the amounts of carbohydrate, protein and fat. What is followed in this book is calories or kilo calories and not food calories. Fixed calories are assigned to each type. One gram of fat would give 9 kcal, one gram of Protein or one gram of

> **Calorie calculation:**
> 100 gram of one type of yoghurt has 7.5 grams of carbohydrate, 4 grams of protein and 0.2 grams of fat. Total calories =(7.5x4 + 4x4 +0.2x9) =47.8 kcals

carbohydrate would give 4 kcal. In the beginning the calculations were done on the basis of the heat the food would produce. The food would be dried to remove water and then the solid was tested in the lab to see how many calories that solid can output. Present method is better than the old method even though not close to near perfect. In the new system the value of animal protein is same as vegetable protein. Protein of each vegetable may give different energy values but considered as same protein. Here just a mass is equated to the calorie. In every calorie calculation, products like vegetable, fruit, nuts, meat or any food is equated like materials. Values stated in calories captured the imagination of the people and people started to read labels and be guided by them. At the same time real energy derived from those different fats, proteins and carbohydrates would vary quite significantly from person to person. Mineral salt or even common salt is not a fat or protein or carbohydrate and can we call that a zero calorie item?

Calories play an important part even though there are lot of assumptions, discrepancies and errors. Some standard helps to compare the products. That is the use of calorie. The energy value one gets depends on so many components that reside in that food product.

The calorie values of 100 grams of few food items are given here for some understanding. With these values one can feel what actual energy would be transferred to the body. Wheat has a value of 340 kcal, rice 356 kcal, cooked rice 130 kcal, white corn 365 kcal, yellow corn 86 kcal, peanut 560 kcal, boiled peanut 320 kcal, dry roasted 584 kcal and meat based on various parts, beef around 160 to 300 kcal, mutton 180 to 240, pork 220 to 540

One day food:
With the energy of one day food a person can walk 2 to 5 kms (1.5 to 3 miles) a day at a speed of 5 to 6 KM/ hour (3 to 4 Miles/ hour

A person can exert around 150 to 200 watts of power at a time. (Guyton, 2006) kcal and chicken 220 to 300 kcal. Water contains so many salt required for our body but has no calories. Salt has no calorie and has its use. The 'no calorie' is as per the system in the food industry due to their inorganic origin. Everything the mind demands and body consumes has a lot of energy and does not depend on the type, size and weight.

The labels in food packets are not uniform. Each company follows their own system and are labelled with the calories for 1 piece, 1 ounce, 1 gram, 1 bowl, 1 tsp, 1 measure, this pack etc. If all the packets are labelled with the number of calories for one gram of food then it would be easy to understand for comparison.

'One man's meat is another man's poison':

This saying is to specify that we are all unique individuals. Dieticians fix the food quantity based on calorie for a patient or for his weight reduction. Lot of research has been done in the assimilation and absorption of various foods. With the reason, that the individualisation of each food with each person for the absorption capacity being difficult and cumbersome, the whole population is generalised. In doing so what the dietician does not know or does not care about is the absorption level in the patient of the diet food that is specified.

Digestion:

Absorption of the food during digestion process is based on individual's digestion and assimilation system. Every food that is consumed by an individual has different absorption capacity. Only if the body is perfect all the calories as per calculation would be absorbed. The vitamins and minerals from natural food would get digested without problem. Organic chemicals of natural compounds would go well with the digestion. Problems happen only when the chemicals like preservatives, colouring agents, etc. present in the food has an effect on the digestion path. These chemicals may not have any calorie but act in the body artificially. The chemicals being artificial it does not go well with the body and gets converted to various products. Not all chemicals, do act with the biological system. Non problematic chemicals would go along the digestion path. Others would get separated to become free. The free ones are the radicals of the compounds and roam around in the body or stays at some specific place. Only antioxidants would help to remove them.

Forced eating creates new health problems due to the resistance the opposing body would give to unwanted food. Digestion would be difficult in this case. Each individual is unique in his digestion system. Assume one person eats and cannot extract that specifics from the food. In that process the required specifics are never acquired into the body. Deficiency still exists. When body works more and more the efficiency of the conversion mechanism goes down. One can observe this with a common salt deficient person by taking more salt again and again. Compared to others in his family one may take more salt and crave for salty food and still may not improve his system. The conversion mechanism goes bad where the salt (sodium chloride) from salt rich food is converted. Because of this aversion in the body mechanism, mind wants to stop the sodium chloride food altogether. What is the reason? This is like love-hate attitude of nature.

Once the love is deep and that is not accepted, hatred starts and reject the love altogether. Same happens with food. The food you like most is not accepted by the body and hatred begins and one day rejects the food altogether. The solution is to repair the mechanism by a medicine.

Weak digestion:

For good health, it is important that the two systems relating to breathing and digestion perform well. One needs energy to breathe and needs breathing to make the energy. Energy is a must for the body functions and the energy resource is the food. The food has to get digested and assimilated to drive the body systems. To operate the digestion machine certain minimum energy is required. If mind is busy in its thoughts, energy for digestion engine may get reduced in certain individuals. After taking the food and even the time you start eating, digestion process starts. If mind activity continues, energy for digestion would be reduced. Hence one feels compelled to have a nap after heavy lunch or dinner. The mind wants to spend full energy for digestion and defer further work after the nap. Else digestion would be delayed or energy output may be less or proper digestion would not happen and some other digestion system trouble would arise. Doctor's advice to the relatives not to pass on any shocking news to an ailing patient is to avoid fainting. When some people get up from the bed suddenly they feel as if light headed with fainting or dizziness. Reason is the same in both instances. During sleep, blood to the brain is less than normal. During the reduced thinking process the blood to the brain is also to a reduced level. One can find the persons who cannot decide or spending lot of hours to make a decision get tired easily. This indicates that the thinking process needs more blood and many parts of the brain works to solve the issues.

The person who resolves the issues fast or decides fast or who has reduced worries need less blood to his head and may not need any nap. The patient who is recovering from his ailments is supposed to spend his energy to cure his illness rather than to waste for his physical and mental activities. Unexpected news or abruptly getting up from bed makes a person to come to the thinking process suddenly with so many events and a sudden rush of blood to the brain. The demand of the brain has to be met in seconds and sudden blood flow up to the brain is difficult when blood has to be diverted from other parts where it was engaged for curing the ailment. If few more seconds are given to the heart, the heart can make up the requisite blood flow. A few seconds makes a difference and the blood cannot be supplied and the system wants you to take rest until the makeup gets ready. This rest is gained by fainting.

Artificial food:

We create lot of food supplements replacing the natural ways of food that used to be from the garden to the mouth. The development in research finding new constituents, new salts and vitamins help the food companies to come up with new food supplements to meet the deficiency in health. One example of salt entry is iodised salt. In analysis it has been found that the Iodine deficiency exists due to the absence of iodine in water. Iodised salts are found to improve and everyone is forced to consume. Iodine deficiency could be targeted after a clear analysis and not every public. Imparting iodine on the specific group would invite new health problems. There are chances for many to get thyroid problems and more health issues due to iodine in excess. This is one example how more health problems enter into even the healthy population. When one food supplement is developed to solve a problem many other problems develop demanding more new products.

Chemicals in FOOD:

Just about a hundred years back we were eating only products of nature. After we started gaining knowledge to manipulate the nature, manmade artificial chemical products started as a part of food. We consume pesticide through milk and fruits. We eat preservatives through packed foods. We enjoy colors with colouring agents in food. We eat TEFLON through the coated utensils. Any material used for cooking, any food derived from chemicals from non-natural resource creates an issue in digestion. When an organic chemical is derived, even if it is from nature, the product loses its value due to its non attachment with the biological system. These chemicals don't go well with the body. Any chemical used in preparing food, unless tested for few generations, are not fit to be used.

Sugar is a chemical, the cause for so many problems of the body, by recent research. The research on sugar is yet to develop. Common food product like sugar, to be avoided or removed from the public, would take time due to the time required in finding replacement which includes business interests.

Nature cannot be controlled by human science. That is the reason modification or destruction is the path followed. Basically we as individuals want to control our family, our relatives, our friends, our surroundings, our garden, our fields, our animals and our environment. The chemicals are controlled by our scientific methods in the industry. What is controlled by the industry can be marketed easily. The mathematical figures and values attract the public which add mental strength for the consumer, as he/she feels he/she is a rational being. With our short experience of few decades, a few who understand the advantages of nature want to go for organic natural products. Others who feel convinced that they enjoy the benefits of the chemical and modified natural plants support the genetic modification process and introduction of artificial food items in the market.

Slow and Fast food:

Speed of the digestion system in our body cannot be increased. Hence we try the fastness in all other external activities. Once, food used to be prepared by slow heating in mud pots and burning wooden logs. Nowadays food is prepared by fast heating. After fast cooking, eating also is fast. Cooking speed increased due to technology development by electricity and petroleum gas. The age old methods of slow cooking by wood and coke are fading away and we cry with the awful effect of fast food. It is difficult to go away from the advanced methods to old methods unless we understand the value of good old slow nature of cooking and the ill-effects of new fast cooking technology. Also technology should be developed for slow cooking. Slow cooking is by reduced heat for long time. Slow cooking adds taste. The energy of the food is not wasted. Compare the energy of raw vegetable and cooked ones. Raw vegetable has high energy than the cooked.

The bad health is not much from fast food, but from fast energy foods like Sugar, Glucose, and Biscuits etc. The major deterioration of health by the medicines is diverted towards the fast food, lack of exercise and sedentary lifestyle etc. The medicines by its side effects make a person weak. When the weak person eats the weak and fast food, health goes down and the fast food is pointed to be the culprit.

Everybody decries the fast food being the root cause and not the fast medicine. The way we eat the food is slowly deteriorating due to the laziness developing in the society. Fruit juice is squeezed for drinking instead of peeling the fruit and eating the pulp. Eating the fruits and vegetables in small pieces is the habit developed not to exercise the muscles in our jaws and mouth. We want to eat small slices of apple and worried about biting and chewing. When biting had stopped, teeth and gums stopped to gain strength from blood circulation and decay sets in. By reducing the effort in biting, eating and chewing we load the stomach with extra work and in one bulk load.

Our body, the product of nature, has not changed in its method of digestion even with all bad inputs through food. We cannot taste fast. We cannot see fast. We cannot smell fast.

Same way digestion cannot be fast. Our body system tries to solve its problems by itself even when an individual eats any food. Just look at the lemon with a temptation and the saliva starts to secrete. The time you start taking the lemon or any food, each part of the body is ready and waiting to work even though its time of work is hours away. Getting ready is essential so that when the food needs the specific items from liver, gall bladder, pancreas, kidney etc. they can deliver for the process of digestion and assimilation. Out of all parts of our body the last one to make a person go down permanently is his kidney. The unwanted chemical of food supplements are extracted through the kidney. Input problems through mouth can be tolerated by our body and not the output issues of solid and water wastes. In this process water plays an important role amongst all food items we consume.

Water:

If a calculation is made for calories the salts in water may add to very meagre value. Plain water as zero calories has no part in adding energy. It looks funny. But that is what mathematics is. Biological calculations are different for the energy that water has and is most important of all.

Bottled water is one of lucrative food item marketed in recent years. In some parts of the world cost of water per litre is higher than the cost of milk. The control of buyer and seller is with the industry is the reason for this. How are we converting normal water to bottled water in order the make it bacteria free, contaminants free and clean? One common method is to heat the water and collect the water vapour and condense to clean water. Natural minerals in water are removed in water treatment by evaporation. This water is clean without any salt or contaminations or sediments. This industrial process removed the natural salts from the water. Then salts are added for taste assuming these are the salts that are required for human health. With our limited knowledge we cleared all natural salts from water by processing it in industry. In that case why we talk of mineral water and water from springs? The natural water from springs passes through soils and plants and collects the minerals in natural form to feed any bio life on earth. Same way water from mountains flowing through different soils and also the rivers collect natural minerals for the basic need of life. There are other processes to treat water. Methods like ozone treatments and RO (reverse osmosis) methods do not spoil the water. Ozone adds energy to the water by imparting oxygen. Do we really know of everything that we need for our body? Yes. We think we know and want to control.

Can we grow more food?

Basic source of our food is from plants and the animals, which eat those plants. Only a little of our food are from salts and minerals. Many salts are through the plant products either grain, pulses, vegetables, fruits or nuts. The scenario changed from a farmer preparing the food product directly from the field to the kitchen. The industry has taken over the job due to population and growing cities. The intention is to get more efficiency from growing plants, getting yields, processing and packing, distributing and selling to meet the in-between costs from the field to the kitchen. If we approach through natural process we have to grow more plants or feed the same plants with more and better manure. Like a human being, plants have limit in its growth. Like humans have a limit in the power output to work plants and animals too have limits in their growth and outputs. Our greed makes us to push the plants and animals to do more than what they could do naturally.

Instead of protecting the plants and using them for our benefits in natural way we try in artificial way to get unexpected advantages. What our scientific inventions tempt us to do is by playing with the science to play with the plants and animals to get what we want. By this way, with our limited knowledge, we want to take control of nature in our hands. Controlling the nature from outside is impossible and hence we want to enter into the core of plants. Our goal looks like 'Cut the hen to take all the eggs in a day instead of waiting and getting one egg per day'.

How we control the plants – Up, down and the basics:

Our thinking is that the animals and plants do not have any brain and they don't have any thinking and have no intelligence or kindness. After trying for so many years to control the plants to grow more grains by fertilisers and increase milk production by artificial feeds our interest has gone deep in all ways to get full control over the organisms that produce food. In case of plants our control is up, down and inside the basics.

Upward we spray chemicals as pesticides to destroy any pest that eats the plant, fruit, bark or leaf or anything. We want the plant to be clean and think the plant would give us the required product. Who created the plant for whom? Every insect and pest has to live on some plants. We are supposed to drive them away and not kill them. By this way human society decimated many animals and plants and also the process is still going on. Whatever insecticide and pesticide we spray on plants come back to our lunch table hiding between the grains, fruits etc. We are happy until we would go sad one day when we realise the ill effects of our deeds but then it may be too late.

Downward we use fertilizers. Also we do not want any other plant to grow nearby thinking that the other plants are weeds. We do not realise that we are growing the plants where the weeds were living for years. This is an invasion by us. Instead of adjusting to live with them we want to destroy all others other than what we want. The fungicides and herbicides find an easy way to come to our dinner table and find a safe place through the vegetables and fruits. We are happy until we would get into troubles.

Basics are the structure of the plant that we are planning to modify. The science has come to a developed state in research where we could decide the nature of the plant from its basics by modifying DNA, called Genetic modification (GM). As an example we want to make the skin of the fruits thick to store for more days than now. So we grow the fruit without seed so that eating is easy, make the seed with DNA modification so that there will be resistance to pests, weeds and disease, more produce with less input. Inject the cows with Bovine Somatotropin (a product to have more yield of milk from the cow) to extract more milk. Genetically Modified food is common nowadays by this type of research. It is said that by this research food problem would be solved. The improved milk through injection from the cow that ate the grass with herbicide and leafs with insecticide finds a way through the bottled milk to the breakfast table. We are happy until we would go miserable one day when we find what has hurt us albeit it is too late to reverse anything.

Using the science is not a problem until we test the products of science. Many fast developments like this are increasing the health problems and we learn of them only after a few decades. After experience of all the chemicals like DDT, Chloroform, antibiotics etc., the GM shall be tested for long time and will take at least a few generations to prove its advantages and ill effects, as this is acting at the core of the human society, the food. Weak biological plants or animals get eliminated and the strong ones survive. When we modify the nature with artificial methods the survival cannot be predicted. Unless we know the biological cycle and prove the tests over generations we should not bet ourselves with nature and take major risks that can affect the fate of our future generations. It has been proven that the plants grown from GM seeds pollinate and change the other normal plants to the GM type (Marsh, 2015).

Simple method to test the good and bad exists in nature. A drop of poison or drop of contaminated water can spoil a pot of normal water. Even a barrel of normal water would become contaminated when added with one cup of contaminated water. Many good ones cannot improve any bad ones. One bad can destroy many.

The energy we get from:

Lowest level species (called trophic level-1 in food chain) have high levels of energy by variety of food contents. The plants and algae are level-1 category and they make their own food by taking nutrients from the soil and energy from sun using photosynthesis or chemosynthesis. The animals eat the plants. The animals absorb energy from plants and the man from animals and plants. That is the reason bottom most organism sustains in the earth compared to top level organisms like animals and plants. Larger and medium Animals are getting extinct faster than insects. Plants stay for long. Many herbs and plants sprout in some corners of the earth even if no rain for years. Plants survive even in deserts and barren lands. When rain or even some moisture wets the land the plants show their smiling face on ground. The plants have reproduction capacity in different ways. Same plant itself has reproduction by its nut, seeds, stem, root etc. Human and animal species have restricted methods for reproduction. How happy the animals and the humans are when they see the plants, bushes, flowers and trees. The food power remains with low level species as food producer than upper species, the consumer. Plants like spirulina, mushrooms, fungi and algae have lot of basic energy components with them. All types of food energy are concentrated in down level species to feed those that are up above. The top level foods like an egg or meat has limited energy.

What we eat has its characteristics embedded in us, grains, greens, nuts or even meat. Natural habits and the availability made us to take food from fertile resources. The food we eat is derived from plants and animals, which has reproduction capabilities. That is the way every animal and plants take the food and reproduce. Nuts, grains, plant parts are fertile and so we are. We are eating food products which have capability to produce seeds. This may be nature's curse that for one to produce seed one should eat plants that can produce seed. What we eat we are that. Our body and our attitude get the characteristics from the food we eat. By looking outside the window or inside the home in the television, we can understand their characteristics and the act of herbivorous and carnivorous animals are based on food they eat. When the grains or nuts are not reproductive we may also not. In case the food is derived from a source of non-productive generation, the destination that consumes may become non-productive. That may be the nature and the way life has been going on for thousands of years. We are not sure of the nature's drama. Experience may show many years later and by that time our ability to reproduce may get reduced. Our advanced knowledge has grown up in the past few decades and that short term ingenuity cannot decide the future and should not destroy the future of mankind unknowingly.

Energized food:

Foods get energy in simple ways. Spring water when it is turbulent with trapped air gets negative ions and the charges become part of water. Water is energized by ozone. Ozone treated water has anti-bacterial property.

Story of water from Ganges - Water of Ganges River is considered sacred. The experience has become a habit to use the river water in all sacred activities. Even though religion is attached to reinforce the belief of the people, the reality is that the Ganges water never decays for long and the tests have proven so.

Ganges water does not decay, rot or putrefy, even after long periods of storage. The British East India Company used only the water from Ganges taken from the Hooghly, one of its dirtiest river mouths, on its ships during the three month journey back to England from India, because it stayed 'sweet and fresh'. When the ships took water from river Thames, it decomposed before they reach to the Cape of Good Hope. Hence they had to refill their tanks entering into some ports of western Africa. The researcher, Hollick's interview with professor of hydrology, DS Bhargava and a Molecular biologist and entrepreneur in Bangalore, Jay Ramachandran revealed the secrets water of Ganges. After investigating water samples by the hydrologist and the biologist it was found that the oxygen levels in the Ganges' water are 25 times higher than any other river in the world, which gives it its self-purifying quality. The high amount of oxygen in the water helps assimilate organic materials, and helpful bacteria destroy harmful bacteria. The water from the Himalayas is from the melting icicles that are oxygenised and the

icicle collection area is large for the river
Ganges (Hollick, 2007).

Even though the nature provides the best quality water in the
river Ganges, we spoil it. That is the man's way to conquer and
to destroy the nature. The important point here is oxygenised
water is the best to use and is anti-bacterial. Doctors advise to
boil the water and drink warm water. By this way you drink
water without energy. Cool the same water. To add energy to
water is to make the water splash mixing with air. The water
fountains in parks and office buildings spread energy around
that area by this way of water mix with air.

Why do we shake the drinks well and mix drinks between
the cups again and again. What do we get there? The water
particles get the energy from air and add taste. Taste is one
which induces the person to drink or eat.

The taste and smell one had in childhood would remain
forever in the memory. For example at the age of five a person
eats a vegetable and liked the taste or the smell but missed
the chance even to see it for many years in between. One day
after 40 years seeing the vegetable would induce the interest.
The information remains embedded in the memory. Mixing
food with a common taste like Tomato ketchup will hide
the taste of basic food. Children should be induced and not
pressurised to eat food of different tastes, which could help
later. The kids, who roam around and eat anything from the
available minimum in villages, are healthier than the children
from cities, who have opportunity to eat anything but never
do (Bjorklund-2010).

Do you know why people advice not to swallow the food
without chewing? The saliva is the energy that mixes with
food. The tribal people and the generation away from cultured
society still use their saliva over the wounds for cure.

Food may have the protein, vitamins etc. unchanged. Body digestion takes care of the energy in the food and easy assimilation. The interest to eat itself adds energy. The eater shall be made to have interest in the food before eating. Fresh vegetables are recommended due to the reason they have energy. Speed of cooking should match with our digestion. Slow cooking collects so many energies from environment to add energy to it. Slow cooking adds the taste. Mud pot cooking gets popularity due to this.

Always bottoms protect and support those at the tops:

Earth and soil supports the small house, heavy structures and tall buildings. Same way nature minerals and plants exist in this earth to protect the higher level organisms like animals and humans. The nature provides us with solutions in the form of herbs, plants and minerals for us to use the intelligence and experience to select and use to get salvation.

Who feeds his body after digestion needs no medicine.

-Thirukkural, a Tamil literature-

8

Medicines

Nature is slow
To us it appears to be dead slow.
Takes for us, humans, 10 months to deliver baby.
Takes 12 whole months to see the next winter.
Takes months for a plant to yield vegetables for our food
Takes years for a tree to deliver its first fruit
Takes anywhere from 24 to 72 hours for us
to digest the food we consume.

But we humans want
things to happen fast
To travel fast by air or by road
Grow the food fast,
Cook the food fast by gas
Cool any food fast by fridge
Heat food fast by microwave
Eat fast to go for work

We want fast paced life
We wish to live long
We wish to get cured fast by consuming the
fast acting medicines.

Nature should match with nature.
How to find right balance between
Nature's speed and
speed of human activities in natural way.

What is medicine?

Medicine is to cure an individual of his ailment. What is cure? Cure means to make the person healthy. The requirement is health and is achieved by clearing out the disease. The basic question to ask here is 'Are we clear about what is disease?' Is the disease the symptoms, the causes or something else? Prime expectation is that the disease should leave the person by consuming a medicine. Basic requirement is to understand the target, the disease. Clearing the disease means to send it away or kill it. The medicine has to do the job. Diseases, as we know them, are theoretical and named after symptoms. Hence we have to deal with the issues that cause the symptoms.

What causes the symptoms? As per common knowledge the germs that cause the diseases are the bacteria and virus. Hence the target is bacteria and virus. The medicine for that disease shall drive them out or eradicate it. Once the symptoms of the disease disappear, it is considered that the person is cured. Is it true? We believe so. Let us see what we do with the bacteria or virus.

Virus can be prevented before it enters into the body. Once it enters the body, it will live its life and no medicine during that period can help to act. Prevention is by immunizations to prevent the attack by virus. The immunizations are made of disease product. These medicines have a reduced effect of a disease. By fighting with the medicine the body prepares the attacking strategy. Next time when virus attacks the body, it has the mechanism to fight and keep the virus away. By this way we are preventing the virus. Bacteria are dealt with in another way. Medicines are given to the patient so that the bacteria are killed or made inactive. Reason is that we have never developed the method for driving them away. How do we kill? We have so many types of pills, capsules and injections that are introduced into the body. Patient waits for the symptoms to disappear.

Else the doctor prescribes another medicine and waits. Person is under medication until the symptoms clear, which is an indication for the cure from disease.

Where from these medicines are derived and manufactured? We may think that all medicines, what is sent into the body are made from herbs. Different medicines are made by the drug industry with the experience of people in taking herbs, plants and mineral salts etc. Gathering this experience, the industry found in the herbs, the technique to extract the chemicals that work to cure the diseases. When demand increased, same chemicals were manufactured by different processes by the pharmaceutical industries with different trade names.

Drugs and medicines:

Pharmaceuticals use the terms drug and the medicines. Public usage is Medicine. A drug is used to make a medicine. Medicine is to cure a patient. Drug is normally taken for pleasure like heroin, marijuana which has an element to incite addiction. Drug, being a substance used in treatment, cure or prevention of disease is the term used commonly in place of medicine. The name, medicine is used, in this book for the medicines and drugs that is being used to cure the diseases.

The medicines are categorized based on its actions on the symptoms except Antibiotics and Antiviral medicines. Antibiotics are for treatment to prevent bacterial infections. Antiviral drugs are to inhibit the development of the virus. The other medicines are based on the symptoms and are many types such as anti-inflammatory for swelling control, antifungal to clear the fungus growth around wounds etc. Other are antipyretics to reduce fever, analgesics as painkillers, anti-malarial drugs for treating malaria, antibiotics for inhibiting germ growth, antiseptics to prevent the growth of germs near the burns, cuts and wounds, mood stabilizers etc.

Hormone replacements are derived from animals. Stimulants, tranquilizers help in many treatments. Various forms of the medicines are tablet, capsules, liquids (mixture, solution or syrup), skin application (creams, lotions or ointments), suppositories (to be inserted into the rectum), drops (for eye, ear, nose), inhalers, injections, implants (patches to be absorbed by the body through the skin), and sublingual (underneath the tongue) medicines. Major medicines are from herbal plants, minerals, substances of marine origin, animal origin and microbial origins. Synthetic drugs are by chemical synthesis, biotechnology genetic-engineering and radioactive substances.

Extended life:

The medical innovation has extended our living years. The breakthroughs were possible by medicines, inoculations, vaccinations, organ replacement, artificial organs, anaesthesia in operations, cultivating nutrition, imparting physical fitness, skin care, hormone medicines, vitamins and the supplements.

The development of medicines was very useful to cure or banish many diseases and helped in containing outbreaks of plagues and other epidemics. They helped in removal of small pox and significant reduction of cholera, malaria, diphtheria, polio, tuberculosis and heart diseases. A person who would have died at the age 47 in 1900 would now live much longer to die at the age of 80 with support of advances in medical field. These ages are average values. A new born in 1900 had life expectancy of 47 years and by 1965 it increased to 65 years. If you examine closely, they are just improvement in numbers, but not living real good quality life, even though this improvement is called the 'Paradox of Medical Progress' (Marmor, 2000).

No doubt there was improvement but day by day the extended age is sustained under medication similar to diabetics. Decades back a person would have lived like a king or queen and gone one day. Now the medicines extended their life to many more years of medication, with daily visits to clinics or bed ridden mostly in hospitals. The extended life is mostly confined to bed and not the full active life that we all desire to have.

At the same time, the diseases have also started developing resistance. These were attributed to the fighting capability of bacteria and virus. This way we have more diseases than before. Old diseases stay with resistance even after development of innumerable types of medicines.

Any medicine that does not cure a disease has no value in the system. In present times, several new medicines have been developed but their efficacy in combating the disease is poor. John Pepper, a theoretical biologist at the National Cancer Institute, says, 'Bacteria are relentlessly evolving resistance and will continue to do so unless we find a different way to fight them. Every time we develop a new drug, it fails" So our approach has been he says "Quick! Make another antibiotic!". With increased cost in developing antibiotics that cut into profits, many pharmaceutical companies started business to target costly diseases like cancer, hepatitis etc. for more profits. Even with the entire crisis above scientists still they try to develop new antibiotics by undertaking a study of age-old experiences of the herbals and practices of remote villagers (Rob Knight-2015).

The medicines are tested with animals like guinea pigs, rats etc., and only then approved for use with the public. Every medicine acts in different ways with different living organism. Each organism has different method of digestion system, disease protection mechanism etc. However this is the system now followed and later researches show even the methods of testing with the animals is a costly affair. Rob Knight (a computational biology pioneer, co-founder of the American

Gut Project and director of the new Microbiome Initiative at the University of California, San Diego) wrote in Scientific American, "The germ-free mice are far too expensive". Increase in cost changes the method of tests of new medicines. Now researchers are trying to move from the mouse model to a test-tube model. Ultimately the move is to a computational model based on DNA sequencing that would be so inexpensive and effectively free. Costly guinea pig would add costs to the medicine and the cheap computations will reduce the cost. Human beings' life that will depend on the medicine is in between! (Rob Knight, 2015).

Short history of medicine:

Medicine has come a long way over the past two millennia. The medicine co-existed wherever man lived. He found the use of everything around himself for his health. The medicine used was made from plants, minerals and animal products. Human food is basically from plants and then animals in everyday life. That is the reason herbs are predominant in the preparation of medicines.

Egyptians would have performed the medical surgery around 2750 BC. A medical record dated to a time as early as 3000 BC was found by Edwin Smith, containing the earliest recorded reference to the brain.

Chinese medicine is from 5th century BC. Traditional Chinese Medicine that is based on the use of herbal medicine, acupuncture, massage and other forms of therapy has been practiced in China for thousands of years and continues with very progressive improvement in health. The wide use of acupuncture is spreading throughout the world due to its effectiveness. Basic Chinese medicine is based on the balance between two subjects, yang and yin like positive and negative, tall and short etc.

Traditional Indian system of medicine is based on three elements that is present in different fluids in the body and their balance leading to health and their imbalance leading to illness. India had three systems of medicines and still we continue to have them namely, Ayurveda (pronounced as Aaayurvaedhaa), Siddha (Siddhaa) and Unani (Unaani) based on the three fluid systems. One of the four age-old Indian scripture called vedas (vaedhaa), namely the Atharvaveda, is a sacred text from early period circa.600 BC, is the first Indian text dealing with medicine. The foundation of Ayurveda has been built mainly on traditional herbal plants. Siddha medicine is a system of traditional medicine originating in Tamil Nadu in South India. Siddha uses variety of herbal plants, minerals and animal products and have different processes to make medicines and these were recorded in the form of verses. Unani got deep roots and royal patronage during the Muslim rule in India and is based on herbs and has similarities with Greek medicine and Ayurvedha.

The oldest Babylonian text on medicine dates back to the Old Babylonian period in the first half of the 2nd millennium BC. The most extensive Babylonian medical text, however, is the Diagnostic Handbook. Arabian medicine had influence from persons like Ibn Sina (Avicenna), who lived in Persia (980-1032), who differentiated meningitis from other neurologic diseases and gave importance to hygiene and holistic approach to the patient. His *al-Qanun fil Tibb* (*The Canon of Medicine*) represented the absolute authority in medicine for over 500 years. Another physician, Ibn-Zuhr (Avenzoar) pointed out the importance of drugs for body and soul. Ibn-Nafis described the pulmonary circulation. Abu al-Qasim al-Zahrawi, 10th century surgeon, wrote the Kitab al-Tasrif, a 30 volume medical encyclopedia. Ibn al-Baytar of Baghdad, in 12th century, wrote most famous manual '*The Comprehensive Book on Materia Medica and Foodstuffs*,' an alphabetical guide.

Homeopathy has roots in Germany by Samuel Hahnemann who in 1796 developed an alternative medicine to the modern medicine called allopathic medicine. This medicine was created based on the principle of 'Like cures like'. A substance that causes the symptoms of a disease in healthy people is supposed to cure similar symptoms in sick people. At one stage Homeopathy was widely used in Europe and US and got reduced in its use after the entry of modern medicine. Homeopathy medicine continues to be used still today in many countries.

Fathers of Western medicine are Galen of Greece (greatest surgeon) and Hippocrates of Greece. The Hippocrates of 5th century had made enormous inputs to the medicine. Corpus is a collection of around seventy early medical works from ancient Greece strongly associated with Hippocrates and his students. Hippocrates invented the earliest oath for physicians, which with significant modifications, is still relevant and in use today.

The principles of Hippocrates are the basis for the modern medicine. Further the germ theory of disease in the 19th century led to cures for many infectious diseases. Germ theory of disease was introduced by the German physician Robert Koch. Pasteur's team added investigations to support the theory. In 1881, Koch reported discovery of the "tubercle bacillus", conforming the germ theory. Medicine was heavily professionalized in the 20th century. The 21st century is characterized by highly advanced research involving numerous fields of science. The mid-20th century was characterized by new biological treatments, such as antibiotics. These advancements, along with developments in chemistry, genetics, and lab technology such as the x-ray and scanning led to modern medicine.

Even though the Greeks were considered the pioneers of medicine they belong to the same genre as the modern medicine, who considered body in the forefront as the diseased part and not the mind. The real forefathers of mind-body system of cure are the Egyptians, Arabs, Chinese and Indians.

What is Modern medicine?

Medicine is to cure a disease. To find a medicine we have to look deep inside between the disease, and the source of disease. Source and reasons are the difficult tasks to penetrate and find. That may be the reason the research started going behind the symptoms, which we see, observe, feel and able to describe. The road we have taken so far, walked, ran, driven and raced may still be far away than the source of the disease. We may have to sit back and think about source and its reasons along with symptoms of the disease that we experienced only after we have failed in all our ammunition and nothing is left out in the case.

Bacteria and Virus:

As per the theory on virus, a patient afflicted with jaundice cannot be treated as the virus has to last its incubation period. Take the example of jaundice, a viral disease. The herbal doctors use the herbs to clear the jaundice within three days. How can they cure a virus in its incubation is a debatable point. Essential in the herbal treatment is food control. One of the herbal medicines prescribed by many doctors in India is an Ayurvedic herbal combination in the absence of allopathic medicine for jaundice. The fact that it does work establishes the fact that there is an inherent contradiction in theories of modern medicine and other older systems.

The modern day medicine system learned to use the active constituents of plants, herbs and minerals etc. However forgot to learn how to administer the cure as was used by the learned tribes and villagers for generations. The experience should have been not only in the material they used but also in the way how it is to be prepared and administered. Modern medicine, in reality is not a medicine or even material from nature, like a plant, an herb, a mineral, an animal product etc. It is extracted from the herbs as a synthetic product or made from other chemicals which mimic the original.

Old and the New:

The time scientific development was progressing with the theory on cells, molecules, elements and atoms the compounds of the herbs had captured the attention of researchers in the medical field. New type of medicines started from factories based on chemicals. After gathering the information on the herbs and what it can cure, the industries had the control on medicines and the fast improvement in the health problems attracted the public attention. The collective and group efforts of scientists and physicians in using the modern methods and technology had interest in using the herbs that were widely used in many countries by previous generations. The data on the herbs and the plants that helped to cure diseases were distributed widely amongst the village doctors and whoever was practising with natural products, or even individuals. They were all having the information in their head as experience and may be with small scribbling notes for their personal use. They had only a little data with them and that too only a few physicians recorded for others to pick up and those were also lost after they were gone.

The wanderers who set on a mission to find new medicine were travelling to every nook and corner of this globe. Sometimes interested individuals helped to find the drugs. Lot of efforts were needed collecting bits and pieces of information from the population based on the interest of the drug manufacturer and his skills to extract information. Soon, in due course of time the doctors and their medical associations had control over the medicines for their approval. By introduction of new medicines, day by day the old herbal doctors lost their patients and their livelihood was affected. At the same time the doctors started neglecting the old system of medicine and advised people against the treatment by herbal doctors, though they were the source of information on herbal pants and cures to develop modern day medicine. By time, the medicine industry gained complete control of the medicines sold in the market for public consumption and profited out of them.

Due to easy availability of medicines and their speedy actions to cure the health problems, people migrated towards the use of new industrial products and deserted the herbal doctors. The herbal healers themselves felt attracted by speedy cure and started prescribing them.

Within the few decades of using new medicines and their improvement, diseases started to increase again sending people to search for new medicines as vicious cycle. Instead of finding the reason for the ineffectiveness of medicines to cure, new medicines are entering day by day into the medical field. Resistance developed by bacteria, side effects of medicines and the result of side effects are wide spread amongst population now. What the medicine seekers and in turn the industry has learned from the age old herbal doctors and also from the fore-fathers of medicine is only about the herb and what it can cure. How come a medicine when used by the so-called 'uneducated' doctors for so many centuries worked for curing the disease whereas it refuses to work now for the drug companies? This uncomfortable question was never addressed or answered.

The well known secret that was not collected in many areas was in which way the herb had to be prepared for administering to the patient. Apart from all the details, the medicine industry never realised that the herbal plant is important and not just the chemicals. The herbal doctors were using only the herbs for years from the time of their forefathers and not any chemical product. The herbs work even now on some population somewhere in remote corners, where modern medicine did not percolate yet, untouched by present day civilization. Herb, meant here is not the type of plant, but all plant materials that could help the health.

Two major points to be noted here are

- The medicine should be a natural product
- The herb to be treated to become a medicine for cure.

How a medicine should to be:

Below are the subjects you face in meets, hearsays, talks, listening, viewing, discussions, observations, resolutions etc. What do the items listed below do?

- A simple look, intent look, kind look, compassionate look,
- Angry stare, fixing eyes on,
- Words, talks, advices, lectures, discussions
- Arrow, bullet, stone,
- Newspaper, leaflets, books
- Audio tapes, music, radio
- A scene on the road, an incident you witness, a video clip, television, movie
- Travel in a bus, car or bike

All the above listed subjects do affect you in some way. The physical objects, that did something in you, have not physically entered into you. After the job is done they go away from your scene, but not from the mind. Where do they go? They hide from you or you hide from them or they stay behind you. Physically they do not enter your body or do not mix with you. Many of the above have effects on you, sometimes modify you, improve you or bring you down also. Also they may go deep inside you. That is the beauty of nature. Medicine shall be like that. Medicine shall affect you and can produce a result in you from the so called disease and shall not mix with you physically. Once its job is done it should get out like any undigested food.

Medicine should be like a soldier. You select and send a soldier to kill the enemy like you send a medicine to kill the bacteria. You give orders. The soldier chooses the weapons and reaches the target, fights, kills and comes back. He comes back with all his limbs intact. He would have lost a bullet and that also may be away on the ground somewhere or inside the enemy's body. Your soldier never merged with your enemy. If he does so, the calamity starts and the purpose to kill the enemy is not achieved and you have lost the battle. Best kill is when the enemy never stands up again and your soldier returns unhampered. If the soldier you dispatch merges with the enemy you send a stronger one to kill both. This continues until you do not see the face of the enemy and his deeds. When the soldiers you sent to kill the enemy merge with them they hide him from you and you have the illusion that the enemy is eradicated. He continues to live sometimes away from your vision with the help of soldiers you dispatched and becomes even stronger with information about your weakness extracted from you by your soldiers.

Take an example of the psychotherapist. He talks with a patient and understands him/her and listens and listens until the patient is satisfied. Then the therapist talks and talks and the problem of the patient disappears slowly. How come? What is the medicine here? How come a discussion with a person with one sided advice with the other just listening to the advice gets satisfied? How can there be a change in attitude, activities, behaviour, manners, relationships and social interactions of the patient?. Does any material transaction happen between the curer and the cured? No.

Medicine shall be a carrier like a soldier. Medicine that goes into the body shall carry something to do the job and should get out unharmed. It should not stay inside, join, mix, blend, intermingle and unify with the body. When the killer and the one to be killed join together, you need to send another medicine to clear the old until the symptoms disappear. These medicines really do not kill but keep the bacteria hidden. The present day chemical medicines merge with you and you take even stronger medicines to make them disappear. Still they hide keeping the enemy, the bacteria, away from your normal perception. You think the enemy is gone but all the chemicals are protecting the bacteria and they themselves are wandering around your body as radicals. To bring the radicals out, you need to send the anti-oxidants and the story continues. The level rises in the basket of disease.

Medicine has to fight the disease killing or driving the germs out and make the disease disappear totally to qualify as a cure. A medicine shall be a carrier without disturbing the system or create new problems and new diseases. Everywhere, a carrier is meant to be person or a material which helps to do the job without involving himself or itself. Medicine shall be the carrier of the energy delivering the same with a force to drive the disease out of the system.

The energy in the material acts as a medicine and not the material itself. Medicine should be like an arrow energized and pointed towards the disease that pierces and kills and comes out. Bullet from the gun penetrates the body, kills and comes out with the same shape. The bullet is same as when entered. What the bullet did? It carried something to kill. Can a bullet in a cartridge do that? No. Energy imparted to the bullet created the force and the energy in the bullet, transferred to the body. The impact on the body made the actual kill. An arrow or a bullet carries the energy to kill.

Can the same medicine work for one disease affecting everybody? That means one type of medicine to cure all persons affected by same disease. What we see here is the symptoms and we decide that the disease is same. The symptoms may be same but the root causes may be different in each due to the different constitution of individuals. The hereditary nature is different from person to person and hence the medicine shall also need to be different for different persons. Not the same arrow can kill all animals or even the same type of animal. Different arrows or bullets will be required for different animals. At times for one type of animal, such as tiger one may need different weapons based on the age, its fierce nature and its physical condition. Each animal or bird needs a different type of arrow or bullet or sometimes different weapon with different design and a different force would be required. Likewise to kill a disease, different medicines are required based on the individual, the character, the physical attributes, the food habits, the symptoms etc.

Many instances have been narrated that many cancer patients even after taking chemotherapy and radiation could not get cured of the disease, but got cured when the individuals had taken a resolve in their mind to weed out the disease. The mind has a big role to play in fighting the disease. Basically what is disease? When body responds in harmony with the mind one feels comfortable. By being comfortable we mean that the mind is at ease. Even if the body has a problem a strong mind overcomes the same and small pain in one's leg disappears once there is a mood to walk. If laziness creeps in, the pain in the leg increases and stays longer.

Any Medicine that has to be used for human beings shall be tested only with humans. Medicine for a dog shall be tested with a dog. A mouse or guinea pig cannot represent a human. The medicine or drug tests are statistical. Statistical Mathematics is the link between number science and natural science. As per science if a medicine is made to cure a disease it should cure all those affected by that disease. But in reality it is not so. The cure is based on natural science for which the statistics is matched.

Yesterday's Medicine is today's poison. Today's medicine may be tomorrow's poison. Within a generation many medicines were proved to be causing problems. A medicine which stays long for a particular disease and works even after decades is the best and most suitable medicine to cure those diseases. Medicine or food established and used over the years by generations without side effects or major problems are the best and suitable for ensuring the health. We follow the old type of food habits to some extent and not the old type of medicines. We are still consuming the same type of food grains that we have been using for generations such as wheat, rice, maize, oil seeds, and vegetables etc. as basic foods. But, in case of medicines we abandoned the old system of herbal cures and found new ones in allopathic cure which have failed us within few decades.

We want medicine to work fast and such medicines are appealing to most people like fast action, fast relief etc. Fast food is recognized lately as bad for health but still the fast medicine is being advertised as very good, for fast relief. For our ill-health we blame fast food and we still prefer the fast acting medicine. Anything which is slow and steady is the one which brings lasting relief and gives strength to the basis of life in all our activities.

Good morning to someone:

Good Morning example... for medicines...

'Good morning' to a visitor written on a placard has little impact compared someone greeting with the same word 'GOOD MORNING'. As a matter of fact, compared to the words from the lips, routine brings one less joy. When you hear the same words from someone close to you with real feelings the effect on the listener is multi-fold.

Medicine should be like a smiling welcome with real feelings saying 'GOOD MORNING'. The feelings transferred and the words spoken disappear in air. No records. But is part of nature, air. The job is done. Word never stays, but its effect on us stays.

Perfect medicine is a combination of word 'GOOD MORNING' when delivered well as a warm greeting. When one knows how to pronounce it with a good feeling to match the listener who hears it in the heart, its effect is tremendous. There is no written word. Once uttered it travels and reaches the receiver with smoothness and disappears imparting a warm feeling from a contented heart. The effect of such greeting is an enabler forming the basis for further discussions in a congenial atmosphere. All feelings of stress between the two disappear and the two persons' minds are receptive for further discourse.

We have with us the Herbs and Minerals as products of nature. They help us to improve our health provided one knows how to put them to proper use. We can make every substance and even manmade substances to work as a medicine with the help of nature that could bring some improvement in real life for everybody.

Aim of medicine is to prevent disease and prolong life.
The ideal of medicine is to eliminate the need of physician.

-William James mayo-

9

Herbs and Minerals

A tree gets its minerals and water
from the soil where ever it lives.
The tree gets what it wants within its limits.
No need to source what is beyond the limit.

An animal gets its food within its reach
where ever it lives.
No need to source what is beyond the limit.

A bird gets its food within its reach
where ever it flies.
No need to source what is beyond the limit.

Humans get the food
from the plants and animals around them
within their reach.
No need to source what is beyond the limit.

Same way medicines should be available and sourced
near or around human habitation

What are Herbs and Minerals?

Herbal plants may be a simple plant, shrub or tree, which has medicinal value apart from its nutrition value. Many herbs have only medicinal values. Minerals are the salts of different types of metals and a familiar example is the common salt, namely the sodium chloride. Here sodium is a metal and chlorine is a gas.

Minerals:

We consume various minerals as required for the body starting from water, day to day food and the mineral supplements. Mineral resource for us is primarily through the grains, vegetables and fruits.

In the modern medicine system, the requirements of minerals are specified as metals and gases. Major contents are calcium, phosphorus, magnesium, sodium, potassium, chloride, and sulphur. Iron, Zinc, Iodine, Selenium, Copper, Manganese, Chromium, Molybdenum and fluoride are minor in content. Very minor are nickel, silicon, vanadium, and cobalt. In our body the metals exist as metallic salts and not as metal. For example sodium exists as sodium chloride, sodium phosphate and sodium sulphate, calcium as calcium phosphate, Calcium fluoride and magnesium as magnesium phosphate etc. The lab results are not done to analyse the salts but to see the metal contents. Hence the bio-chemic test results of blood do not represent the contents of minerals in the body. The prescription is based on the metals assuming that the body will convert one form of metallic salts to another form. Lot of assumptions and statistics guide the physician in the treatment to prescribe these inorganic compounds (Schussler, 1914),

Herbs to modern medicine:

Modern medicine had their origins only from the herbal medicines. The herbs used by different communities throughout the world helped to develop the disease treating products as pharmaceutical drugs. Compared to the crude way of handling of herbals, modern medicine were manufactured with quality control, safe packing, and clear instructions for use and released to the public only after approval from government authorities. The widely distributed knowledge of the herbs of various lands was used in making the medicines. The compounds present in the herbal plants were painstakingly identified and associated to a disease for a cure. Analysis required finding what ailment it treats. Finally the extraction of that component from the herb was carried out in a laboratory and then in a large scale.

When the demand increased and availability of the required quantity of herbs was inadequate, the problem arose as how to produce the required quantity of medicines. Many herbs can grow only in certain terrain and specific climates. Lack of availability in time and in the required quantities induced the pharmaceutical firms to do research to grow the plants in biotechnical way. The medical plants and even the herbs for food supplements were grown adopting techniques such as vitro propagation and genetic transformation to increase the productivity. The limitations in bio-agricultural growth made same compounds by industrial processes also (Chandra -2013).

The development of science and the meagre amount of available herbs was the driver for synthetic chemical production. Also controlling the chemicals is easy than the cultivation, treatment, transport and processing of the herbs.

By this time, the usage of crude medicines was past history in the drug industry. Major medicines were not sourced from herbs. Very few medicines are still extracted from herbs and then purified to meet pharmaceutical standards. Even this small quantity of herbs also may not be continued if the demand increases for the drug and it is found to be cheaper to produce the required chemical component by chemical processing.

Modern Medicine to Herbal:

Use of herbs existed for so many millenniums and the experience from the use of different herbal plants was in vogue around those people for the treatment for the sick. In those days nobody went far away to fetch any herbs for the treatment of their ailments. Local herbs of that region were used as medicine for the people of that locality. Use of herbs is still wide spread in many countries where the modern medicine finds it difficult to enter or where the modern medicine is costlier than the local medicines or where the people realised the importance of the herbal medicines after experiencing ill-effects of the modern medicine

Use of herbal medicines is slowly increasing even in the developed countries of American and European continents. Many East Asian countries, China, India, African countries use herbal medicines even though some of the old herbal preparations are decaying. After the experience of modern medicine and its ill-effects, the herbal doctors are back, tracking the herbal preparations and even industries started making herbal based products. Many of the industrial products are just herbals without much medicinal values. Only the herbs with medicinal effects would work towards cure. Else would act as special foods.

Basic herb:

An herb is a plant that is used only when required to resolve a health problem. Some herbs are used in normal food also. The herbs have some characteristics in improving certain systems of the body or rectifying some problems of the person. An herb is like a specialist among the physicians, the food plants.

Herbs are used for food (culinary), flavouring, aromatics (perfumes) and medicines. Herbs like basil, parsley, and thyme are used as foods and in cooking. Herbs regularly used in food are distinguished from the ones that add flavours to the food. The spices add flavour apart from its medical inputs to the food. The smell and taste is an import part in eating and digestion. The spices do that job even in small quantities. The herbs used in cooking for flavour are derived from the small plants and big trees such as leafs (green mostly in cooking and dried as spices), flowers, seeds, bark, roots and fruits. Some typical products like ginger is used in food when green and when dried it gets a medicinal value. Herbs used as perfumes induce a sensation, mood and feelings, which helps for mental uplift.

Even though the industry started finding the so called useful chemicals from the herbs and may find even more in future, the use of herbs in its natural form did not exist. The natural form has advantages and not the chemically converted form. How come when the crude herbs used directly by the village doctors to treat same disease for so many years cannot be cured by the same herb by the industry is big question? The reason is the industry started making the chemicals out of herbs and not the herbs themselves.

Herbal treatment:

Use of the herbs depends on the experience of the herbal doctor, the type of cases he treats and the medicines he uses for long. The cure lies on the doctor's observation, decoding and the medicine selection. Normally herbs are not consumed as a crude herb. Some take the herbs as medicines just as a raw item also. It works as a food and the person gets well too. Herbs are treated to gain energy to have power to penetrate in the system to drive out the bad condition of the body.

Herbal Remedies are prepared in several methods, in different forms and stored for long use in different ways. The methods are grinding, mixing with other herbs, boiling with water or oil, extraction or addition of similar herbs. Grinding between stones or boiling with different mixtures is important activity for most of the herbs. The preparation methods convert the herb to a medicine adding force, vigour and dynamism. Same herbs have diverse healing powers in different methods of preparations and different forms. The forms in which the preparations made are powders, pastes, ointments, poultices (heated medicinal substance on a cloth), salves (creams for wounds), liquids, oil mixtures, infusions (hot teas with herbs), decoctions (extraction from boiled preparations) and tinctures (using alcohol, oil or water extracts). Sometimes one stage is not sufficient and multiple stage and treatments may be required. Adding some more herbals and processing of new compounds are practiced nowadays. The preparations are stored for short time or long periods. To store for long time the medicine is normally stored mixed with oils, alcohols or any other medium which would act as a carrier without affecting the character of the medicine.

An experience with a village doctor:

An herbal doctor was asked to give treatment for a menstrual problem of a girl. The doctor listened to the patient's problems and finally asked whether she attained the puberty and she replied 'No'. The doctor suggested to those, who accompanied the girl, using the leaf from a plant that is yet to bloom. Then he explained from which part of the plant the patient shall pick the leaf and how to grind and use the leaf of the plant.

The point here is a leaf from a plant, which started blooming, has a difference from the herbal plant which is yet to flower.

Herbal treatment takes five stages and each stage is significant in deciding a match between the patient and the medicine. Case observation, herbs selection and collection, preparation, how to take in and duration of treatment are the five stages. Even though the basic steps involved are normal, the method of handling the sick, medicine preparations and how the sick is treated varies from place to place and person to person.

First thing the herbal doctors do is to ask the patient to wait. While attending to other patients who came earlier, this patient is also observed to understand about his nature, attitude and his sickness. Not all the week days a doctor would treat the patients. Specific timings and days of the week are considered important. Morning or evening, Full moon and new moon days are somewhat special for treatment. The herb and its final product will be decided after discussion with the patient. Normally herbal doctors listen more than they talk.

Second is the herb collection. The doctor may have with him some herbs or he has to collect a fresh one. Some doctors request the patient to collect what is required. There are lot of intricacies in collecting a simple leaf from plant, Season, summer or winter, moon times (waxing or waning moon), time of the day, growth level of the tree etc. In few cases the type of herb depends on the person, his ailment, age and his disease state. The boxed text on *'An experience with a village doctor'* is an experience for a simple typical case. One herbal plant does not mean it is to cure only one disease. Also mix of many herbals may be needed for a cure. Different parts of same plant, the leaf, bark, flower, root of same herb may be used for different ailments. Each has different characteristics in their actions.

Third is the preparation. Some herbs chosen shall be green and fresh from the plant and the medicine will be made fresh. Some can be stored for a long time after drying in the sun or in shadow. Many doctors use the medicines already available with them. If preparation takes time, the patient will be requested to attend on some other day. The medicine making process is very elaborate and important and need careful supervision. Once the final medicine to consume is derived and ready, instructions will be given to the patient on how to consume.

The fourth is how the patient has to use the medicine. Patients are advised to take the preparations directly with a specified amount or through a medium like honey, oil, milk etc. Most of the herbal medicines are taken in empty stomach like an hour before or after food, which is different from modern medicine. The modern medicine is volume based and should mix with food for absorption, where as herbal preparations are effect based with a small volume and to be absorbed from the sensory organs (mouth, tongue, nose and skin) and absorption is better before the stomach starts its digestion process. There is restriction, during the medication, that certain food items shall not be consumed.

The Fifth level is the duration of medication. The intake may be daily or weekly and the duration may vary from days to months. Each herbal doctor has his/her own method for the dosage and duration based on the disease, medicine and the person. Normally medicine is taken for a long time for a chronic problem. The basic fact is improvement of health is slow by herbal medicines. Some individuals show an improvement only after few months. Everything is a slow process starting with medicine and its actions and at the same time it is a steady progress.

Herbal medicines are not only given to the ailing patients but at times also to normal persons who want to improve their health. The purpose is to keep the body healthy to avoid any future onset of disease. The herbal medicines can help to build a person's resistance so as not to face major sickness.

Sacred herbs - Some societies consider some of the herbs as sacred. Sacred herbs are due to manmade ingenuity, created by our forefathers for the welfare of their future generation. They made it sacred so that the public will use in everyday life considering as important as medicine so that every individual would benefit. These plants would find a place in every occasion in the family or in the community. Such herbs are Turmeric, basil, frankincense, myrrh, ague root, white sage, cedar etc. Each community uses these herbs in different occasions.

Multipurpose herbs with few examples – Onion are available as so many varieties. The shallot (Allium cepa var. aggregatum) small red onion variety in south East Asia is used for reducing blood pressure (with names, bawang merah kecil in Malay, brambang in Indonesia and in India the names for shallots are kanda, gandana, pyaaz, gundhun, cheriya ulli, chuvanna ulli, chinna ullipayi or chinna vengayam). Garlic and Onion along with Turmeric is common ingredient in Indian foods. Garlic is special for any stomach troubles. Neem (Azadirachta indica) is something special in Indian life and used from childhood problems to preparations of insecticide in agriculture. These are considered having multiple personalities. Cooking specials with medicinal qualities are the herbs Basil, Parsley, Thyme, Rosemary, Sage and Mint.

Who adds taste?

When tea is prepared using tea bags dipped in hot water and mixing them and drinking it, one cannot enjoy the tea due to its poor taste. But a coffee from a coffee machine makes a big difference. Just prepare a coffee or cappuccino and inject steam into it. The foam that is created adds an instinct to drink with a positive feeling. If you have interest use the same coffee with foam and exchange the coffee between two cups mixing them as if coffee pours like tap water from one cup to the other. Do it four to five times. The waterfall effect you created adds a taste to the coffee.

One can find this type of mixing of the tea cup to cup in small tea shops in streets and Indian restaurants but not in restaurants of big hotels. The small shops add a good taste to the tea by their actions to whip up the froth without adding anything materially.

Medicine is not only a science; it is also an art.
It does not consist of compounding pills and plasters;
it deals with the very processes of life,
which must be understood before they may be guided.

-Paracelsus-

10

Chemicals

We have fresh fruit from trees
We drink packed, coloured and preserved drink

We have flowers and plants in nature
We decorate homes with synthetic plastic flower pots

We have forest
We visit to see the animals in the zoo

We have earth
We aspire to go to the moon and Mars

We have feet
We want to travel by cars

We have herbs from nature
We consume synthetic chemicals as medicines

Chemical world:

The herbs were used for centuries and the new modern science within few decades brought the chemicals as medicine and as additives to many food products. Going back to our old food items and habits is not that easy as we so easily forsake our age-old skills and practices due to the technical advancements. People of current generation would not even recognize how a natural food product would look like. The society gets into troubles within a short period by the use of chemicals in all fields of life. The chemicals that affect our health directly are more in the field of medicine and food. Medicine is direct chemical in our intake and the food we consume is embedded with chemicals from so many resources.

Chemicals in Food:

One may ask. We grow the food we eat. Why should we worry? Food cultivation is not under your control. That is the main worry. It is true that your food is not going to be perfect even if you are away from the modern society by thousands of kilometres in a remote land. You get chemicals into the system somehow while growing food, treating the food and eating the food. Even if you are in a far off land what might affect the food crop are the soil and the sky. Water in the land from a river or even sub soil water flow carries something from somewhere like pesticides somebody used in his land in a location upstream. When somebody somewhere tests a nuclear device even thousands of kilometres away, it does not mean you will be spared from troubles due to radiation fall-out. Somewhere somebody pollutes the air by petrochemical products or exhaust gases from processing industries or power houses using coal. You have been cursed to taste or imbibe everything for free and later-on pay to the disease cleaners and health improvers.

What is added to the food in the industry are food-grade chemicals, processing aids, flavoring agents (to add enticing smells), vitamins (to rectify deficiencies), Emulsifiers (to extend the storage life), sweeteners (substitute for sugar), color additives (for appealing colors to attract kids and even adults), and functional food ingredients. While some additives are harmless, many cause everything from simple skin rashes and asthma to vomiting and headaches in some people. Suggestions by naturalists are to avoid foods with synthetic ingredients but to purchase foods that contain natural additives in fruits and vegetables.

Some innovative methods in business have spoilt the natural element in the products from the agricultural fields. Many interesting industrial treatments are used to store the garden products for long time and by that way spoiling its healthy nature. METHYLCYCLOPROPENE is a gas and is used to slow down the ripening of fruits like apple. This gas also is used to help maintain the freshness of the garden flowers. The gas, Sulphur dioxide, serves to reduce the ripening of grapes. Imitation vanilla flavorings are made from petroleum or paper-mill waste. Aspartame is a sugar substitute and is sold commercially and was hailed as a savior for dieters, who did not like the unpleasant taste of saccharin. Later aspartame has been proved to cause problems ranging from allergies and premature births to liver damage and cancer. Benzoic and Sodium Benzoate are often added to milk and meat products as preservatives and also in many foods, including drinks, low-sugar products, cereals and meats. Both are known to cause headaches, stomach upset, asthma attacks etc. Butylated hydroxyanisole (BHA) and Butylated hydroxytoluene are added as a preservative and to delay the decay, the rancidity in oil-containing foods. The World Health Organization's (WHO) International Agency for Research on Cancer considers BHA a possible human carcinogen. Monosodium Glutamate (MSG), which is added in many processed food products is believed to cause tightening in the chest, headaches and a burning sensation in the neck and forearms (Dr. Mercola, 2009). Potassium bromate is used to increase the volume in white flour, breads and rolls. Potassium bromate is known to cause cancer in animals and an even small amount in bread carries a risk for humans. Sodium Nitrite and Sodium Nitrate is in use for centuries to preserve meat. Sodium nitrite combines with naturally present amines in the meat to form carcinogenic compounds. A study by the Cancer Research Center of Hawaii and the University of Southern California suggests a link between eating processed meats and cancer risk with a higher risk of pancreatic cancer. Sodium nitrate can increase the risk of developing heart disease by damaging the blood vessels. (Coupon Sherpa, 2010).

Food is a chemical:

We worry if there are additives in the food that may create health problems. If one major food item itself is a chemical how do we feel? In 1968 Procter & Gamble researchers synthesized a fat substitute called sucrose polyester. Olestra is its name. Olestra is sucrose (table sugar) molecules which are esterified to many fatty-acid residues. Like fats and shortening, olestra is used to fry foods. Olestra may cause abdominal cramping and loose stools (anal leakage) and inhibits the absorption of some vitamins and other nutrients. Olestra is derived from sugar and is considered an additive. Food derivative causing a health problem as observed has a great impact. Is sugar itself is a problem? We do not think so because we assume that sugar is a natural food. The chemical in food is one part. To get a treatment due to the effects of food chemicals your approach to a doctor is another part. Again you are prescribed with another type of chemicals.

A prescription and the chemical effects:

The prescription is written normally with four medicines for an average case. A typical case is explained here. The physician prescribes the first one as the main medicine and this is supposed to work and cure. Main medicine is for the disease based on the ailment and pathology. However the main medicine would have side effects like vomiting, digestion problem etc. This has to be avoided, else the patient would be afraid and this would complicate the case. The patient's attention will be diverted to other health issues. The second tablet or capsule is to nullify the side effects of the first prescription. Side effects from second medicine would be more tolerable. Both the first and the second even if they work perfectly, it is going to act as expected of any chemicals and some of the products from these two medicines will disintegrate and escape from the main medicine. The chemical reactions are so much and some free molecules would be formed. Here surfaces the added necessity to catch the free radicals. The third is an anti-oxidant to clear the radicals of the medicines that will spread or accumulate in the body part somewhere. Body has to cope with all the three artificial medicines prescribed and body would lose the energy. Hence a vitamin or multivitamins or combination of minerals etc. would be prescribed as the fourth to take care of the weakness induced in the body condition.

Antioxidant:

Above was an explanation for an optimum prescription in modern medicine. The important point to note here is the antioxidant to bring the radical out from the body. What for are the antioxidants and what purpose do they serve in the body mechanism? This is like someone goes missing in the battle field and we are sending some specialist to retrieve him back. Some fighters leave the fighting scene and they should be searched and brought out of the battle field, or their bodies.

With all the science and advancement in knowledge and the scientific data available, we could still not master our battle field within the human body. We send the specialists like anti oxidants to do that job. We are not clear which radical is inside and which anti oxidant can bring it out.

They are the free radicals (See the text box). Study of radical is an important subject in the field of medicines. Medicine when consumed could not be absorbed in the digestion system. Some substances even when not digested will not be secreted out of the body. Some compounds may get oxidised and get separated from main compound and become free. The free radicals by chain reaction would form more free radicals. The chain reaction would damage and cause the death to the cells.

> **Radical and Antioxidant:**
>
> Radical is free compound not under any control. A free radical would wander anywhere inside the body system and would create nuisance. Radicals are formed when they are oxidised. Oxidation means losing electrons from its orbits.
>
> Radical is thief and Antioxidant is a cop.
>
> Antioxidant is to clear the radicals. Purpose of Antioxidant is to grab the radical and fetch it out. Antioxidants having extra electrons will recover the radicals from the body to be expelled through the body outlets.

The radical in the society are similar to the same formed in the body. Radicals in our society are the people who do not have any attachment with anybody and roam

Good Morning example:

Modern medicine is like a word 'GOOD MORNING' with jumbled
letters out of sequence. When one knows the language he can find the
word combining the letters. When the chemical matches and assembles
well in the body there is some use and it helps to fight the disease else
the chemicals, being not natural does not go well with body and trashed
away as radicals. The letters of the word 'GOOD MORNING' too
conveys no meaning when written as 'OOM RING ONGD'.

around freely. They are the culprits among the public and they
remain mingled with the public. They are not bound by the
norms of responsible civil or social behaviour and are free from
controls of the society or their families or their friends or other
people around. Even they adversely influence their friends to
turn out as radicals and spoil the society.

An antioxidant can help to absorb the radical. Many vegetables
and fruits are good antioxidants and help to improve the health
by clearing free radicals from human body. Physicians also
prescribe the antioxidants based on other medicines. The
antioxidants react with those compounds and would form a
biological compound and would find a way to be excreted out.
In some cases even antioxidants cannot remove the radicals
from the body. Each antioxidant has its own property and
taking another antioxidant as chemical would lead to another
oxidation problem. Antioxidants in natural form may help to
combat with the situation to some extent. The analogy to this
is like creating a thief and letting him loose to wander and then
attempting to capture him.

Modern medicine is usually a combination of one or more
chemicals. One disease should be treatable by one or more
medicines and in course of time, we should come to a stage
that a specific medicine is meant as cure for a specific disease

and stay that way forever. Some improvements to same medicine are acceptable. But in reality, as seen currently what does the development of new medicines for the very same disease indicate? At least for simple ailments such as fever and cold, one would expect that the right medicine should have been found and established as cure. Even for a simple fever no medicine is found for a positive cure. There is stability in all the areas of science except the medical field and in the field of computers and programming. Change, as part of technical advancement in any field, is acceptable. The basics and fundamentals shall be stabilised. In these fields Basement is weak and building is made strong.

Acute problems even though have links with heredity is more connected with the day to day situations based on environment and the surrounding situations, contacts and food issues. Many herbal doctors give medicines based on disease. One can find that some local doctors are specialised in a particular type of diseases and few to cover overall health of a person. Some doctors analyse in detail and issue medicines. Chronic diseases have main base with heredity and the individualised analysis of a person for finding a medicine should be the future.

Many tribes have used the same leaf or bark for centuries for curing a health problem. They are stabilised and definitely cure the disease. Modern medicine should have brought those barks and leafs in a proper format and used them for curing the illness. The chemicals synthesised out of that bark or leaf could never solve the problem and at the same time the earlier method of cure using directly the bark and leaf has also disappeared with the older generation of people. The newer generation of people lacked the faith and trust in the older system of cure, who discarded the old systems as unscientific and lacking scientific validity as effective cure. Sadly, today there is no place to search for the old grandmother's medicines except in our own back yards only if one should care to find.

The chemical medicines create an apparent improvement in the body when one takes medicines. Patient never feels the disease lurking inside his body. Some disease reappears after few years or if it is too late, the patient succumbs to some disease. The chemicals imbibed into the system create new problems and named as new diseases. Take for example of penicillin (penicillin V), which was used widely and cured lot of cases some decades ago. World War II used this antibiotic to a large extent. Four years after drug companies began mass-producing penicillin in 1943, microbes began appearing that could resist it. The first bug to battle penicillin was Staphylococcus aureus. This bacterium is often a harmless passenger in the human body, but it can cause illness, such as pneumonia or toxic shock syndrome, when it overgrows or produces a toxin.

Penicillin has lot of side effects. By long term use many allergic reactions are possible like difficulty in breathing, swelling of face, lips, tongue, or throat. Serious side effects are diarrhoea that is watery or bloody, fever, chills, body aches, flu symptoms, easy bruising, bleeding, severe skin rash, itching, peeling, unusual weakness, reduced or no urination, agitation, confusion, strange thoughts, unusual behaviour, seizures, convulsions. Few of the problems with reduced seriousness are nausea, vomiting, stomach pain, vaginal itching or discharge, headache, swollen or black coloured and hairy feel tongue, white patches inside the mouth or throat. The list is not complete.

Apart from its side effects a lot of consideration is required about the persons' compatibility with other medicines, while making a prescription. Many reactions are expected and test dose is given to check those allergy problems. After all these problems with penicillin its requirement exists even now. Reason is penicillin has capability to deal with multiple diseases as compared to other antibiotics.

Side effects:

By taking more of antibiotics, the resistance developed in the body and the acceptance of the antibiotic in the system poses a problem. The medicine has to find a way to get out of the body and when it eventually gets out it causes disturbance to so many systems, which we call as side effects. Most of the medicines cause side effects due to its non-natural characteristic.

Bacteria and disease:

Robert Koch found the bacteria, which causes cholera. To test the working of the bacteria Patten Koffer and his assistant had taken the bacteria. One had the cholera disease and another did not. Matchim Koff of Paris along with his friends subjected themselves by taking bacteria of the cholera. Though 12 persons took the bacteria only one got the cholera. This was a proof that bacteria need not affect everybody even when they are attacked. So many factors are hidden to us. Until then there is no logic and only statistics.

Medical world and also the world of nature are not logical but statistical. Statistics link the logical sciences, physics and chemistry with the life sciences. Maths is invented science and is manmade and hence is always perfect and obeys all laws of mathematics. Hence mathematics is easy to manage. Organics are difficult to manage as they are governed by nature. In the same way chemicals are easy to be managed in lab and industry as they are separated from organics. Hence medical research found the easy way to do research in chemicals to find medicines. The disease is part of nature and the chemicals are not part of nature and hence do not match in their functions when they work together.

Experience shows that the herbs and plants do not disturb the body contrary to chemical medicines. Reason is that they are products of nature. The chemicals and the body do not have a matching speed and alignment. Chemicals can also carry the force and serve as cure if it does the job and leaves the body. Even the natural products should not be used in its basic form to drive out a disease. All products of medicine shall be applied like a bullet carrying energy, like an arrow with a force, like a word that has an impact on a person, like a speech that could change one's life and like a rocket that goes out of earth. They have energy to act and same way energized medicines would act without leaving any traces behind.

"The saddest aspect of life right now is that science gathers knowledge faster than society gathers wisdom."

-Isaac Asimov-

11

Energy in Medicine

A verbal command has no value unless
delivered with the right tone.
An arrow cannot pierce
unless it is shot out of a bow with force
A bullet cannot hit the target
unless it is fired from the pistol
A ball cannot fly
unless kicked with force
A wheel cannot roll
unless pushed

One cannot improve his work
without motivation

All have energy but latent energy
which is static energy
but
need dynamic energy
having the force
for an action to occur.

Material cannot work
on our systems
unless
it is triggered

Two patients – two doctors:

A patient enters the consultation room of the doctor. Doctor asks 'what is the problem'. Patient talks and Doctor listens. He waits for the patient to complete his narration and then asks a few questions to clear his understanding. 5 minutes. Doctor thinks for a while and prescribes some lab tests and medicines. The doctor advises the patient to see him next time with test results. Within those five minutes of interaction and viewing the

> **Another patient:**
>
> A patient enters the room of the doctor. The Doctor asks 'what is the problem'. Patient starts and before he/she could complete the doctor says 'I understand'. Doctor thinks for a while and prescribes some lab tests and medicines.
>
> The doctor advises the patient to see him next time with test results. Same 5 minutes.The patient returns home worried after seeing the expression in the face of doctor.

smiling face of the doctor, already the patient starts feeling better and half of the disease has already gone! The patient collects the medicine and returns home with a happy face. Without consuming any medicine how could he/she feel that disease is leaving? The satisfaction. Is the satisfaction a medicine? Yes. Some doctors know it and know how to use it. The text box 'Another patient' briefs the reactions of another patient with a different physician.

Pressure of mind and relief of pain:

Many persons feel like narrating an incident or event or a discussion to someone close to them or even to strangers. They do not and cannot keep details of certain incidents with them. The reason is that sharing the details of such events brings relief to the individuals. Mind feels relaxed. This is like steam pressure venting out of a pressure cooker. Mind gets perturbed by some events. Venting the mind by narration to others takes off the pressure and cools the mind. The pressure due to the event on the mind creates disease symptoms in some individuals. Some persons never get pressure by such events and they face no problem. Just as the pressure needs to be released for protection of the cooker, the individual could suffer health issues if he did not vent out his mind to someone.

Disease in our system:

Disease is like a waste basket. However, as a matter of fact, it is not so simple to clear this disease basket unlike a waste basket. It is of course ideal for all of us to have an empty basket and be free of health problems. What we achieve by using some medicines is similar to covering the top of the smelling basket with some perfumed papers. We feel satisfied for a while thinking we have no more the disease. Same as disease, residual toxins from medicines, chemicals from food in our body and cannot be completely eliminated by the digestion system. This leads us to imagine that we have so many diseases. We have so many symptoms and all belong to one disease basket. Only one disease in a person could give an impression from its symptoms as if he has multiple diseases like many dirty items having different type of smells permeating the air around a waste bin. One person with one disease basket is the most common case. Some persons could have more than one. The first basket is of the diseased body and can be under control of the individual. The second basket is of the mental disorder is not under that person's command. Somebody close to the person has to clear the second basket of disease and only then he can tackle the first basket.

Purpose is to clear the present problems and avoid the future inconveniences. Building a resistance to the body and stabilisation of the mind would help avert future maladies. But we have to tackle the present malady first. By the time the present problems are cleared a positive feeling and confidence develops in the person building up the strength of mind and body.

A medicine has to clear the defects of the heredity, repair the mechanisms and improve the efficiency wherever deficient and clear the disease products of the heredity and toxins. The troubles in some mechanisms may be due to the toxins in the system also. Over all we can see two types of problems. One is the deficiency in mechanisms meant for converting the input to the requirement of body. The inputs may be from all senses of feeling, seeing, smelling, eating and tasting. The second is the toxins that stagnate inside. Toxins may enter the system from outside or created by the bad actions of the mechanisms. Our body systems should be developed such that it rejects the toxins and eliminates or ignores it and be immune from it. In such a case, even if toxin enters the body it would get out without troubling the body. Even the attitudes of the person which are toxins of the mind are important to be cleared from the body. This may appear to be an ideal goal and tough to reach but as much as succeed in staying close to the ideal we benefit from a near perfect health.

Method to deal:

Disease is like an enemy, whom you do not want to be as a part of you. Should you kill the enemy or just keep him at bay? You can live in peace so long as the enemy stays away from you and has his own life without disturbing you. Slowly you forget him and erase thoughts of him from memory unless he would resurface somewhere in the corner. Same way the purpose is served to drive the bad live elements from your

> **How to deal with roach:**
>
> Try one simple method. Kill a roach and leave the dead where cockroaches frequently roam around. You don't find them until the smell of the dead roach stays around for few days. You do not smell the roach but the roaches do.

body and not necessarily by killing them. Let us see which would be the best option, killing or creating a fear to drive away the unwanted. When you kill a fly with a fly-swat you wait for the next fly to be killed. You go on killing as it occupies your mind. Take a roach for example, you keep bait and kill. You become habituated to keep the bait daily. The roach develops a resistance to the bait, just as the bacterium develops its power to deal with antibiotics. The bait you buy after few trials needs to be stronger, the reason being the insects have learnt by now, how to fight and resist.

There is some basic concept briefed in "How to deal with roach" (see the text box). Only by experimentation we will get convinced. The roaches do not like the smell of their own body. Why? Animals, we Homo sapiens, insects, birds also cannot tolerate and be near the cadaver of the same species. There may be exceptions but a few. In the bio systems, only the plants can take the energy and food from their decayed parts in soil.

We humans are building our homes, tilling our lands, constructing the factories where the vegetation once lived and insects, pests and animals roamed freely and enjoyed as it was their natural habitat for over thousands of years. Out intrusion has replaced the homes of several species. Many are already facing extinction and now we make fresh campaigns to preserve those after having been the root cause for their annihilation. We feel that we need them now as they are a part of the evolution chain. We repent after causing their devastation. What has been wiped out of earth cannot come back alive. At least with the existing organisms we should learn to co-exist. Our aim in modern medicine is to make the bacteria dead or inactive. What we should try and do is to have the bacteria but inactive unable to penetrate and harm our health. In the past, we tried to eradicate bacteria and virus by so many drugs to drive them out and those drugs have caused us more harm to our systems. Best approach should be to drive the disease causing entities, whatever it is, out of the body systems and again strengthen the body's defence so as to keep them at bay so that they do not re-enter the body. The Chinese recognized this fact for long, as their saying 'Yin-Yang', which is based on opposites, will always coexist and shall be in balance.

Learning from a farmer:

A farmer, native of southern India, was struggling to solve the problem of rats in a rice field for a long time. Later he experimented a solution to keep the rats away.

> The rice fields of the farmer were infested with rats just before the harvest and started spoiling the grains and making holes in irrigation canal bunds creating unnecessary water drain too. Also snakes started coming to paddy fields to feed on the rats and the farmer walking in the fields felt unsafe. What the farmer did was to catch two rats using a rat trap. Killed them both and put inside a closed pot with water, sealed and kept in storage for a few days for the carcass to rot and disintegrate. Once the rats got decayed fully, he used a cloth and squeezed out the foul smelling extract. Then he added some more water and made a thorough mixture, which he then sprayed along the bunds where the rat holes existed. From the next day he could not see any rats or snakes and he could harvest the rice in a few weeks without any further damage (Pon Sivar-2013).

In a similar pattern, if you look at the wars and battle fields of the past, army of Elephants faced elephant army, horse with horse, sword with sword, bow and arrow with arrow and bow and soldier to soldier. This is similar to inoculations for virus but in a different way. To counter attack one subject use a like subject with a greater force is the norm to succeed.

What is Energy and how can that be used in medicine:

As explained before, compare a bullet carrying energy and an arrow carrying energy. By this way, any material our body is able to take in as a natural organic product can be used as carrier like an arrow or bullet. The energy has the power to make the organic product travel and act with the target. Arrow carries the energy with its own property. Bullet carries its property. When you want to deal with somebody you talk to him as equal and sometimes even more, but in his language so that he understands. Only like subjects can deal with and resolve issues effectively.

Cumin seed energized:

Drop 4 or 5 grains of cumin seed in one litre of water and boil the water to make 200 ml with slow heat. It may take more than 30 minutes. Then cool the water and preserve.

Next morning make 3 parts and drink early morning, mid day one hour before food and night after food. Cumin seed is likely to clean the stomach. What acts now in the bio system of the body is the energized water by the Cumin seed and few the particles of Cumin seed.

A sample way to energize:

A sample method in Indian system is to use a common food ingredient used in cooking to make a medicine for digestion problems. Cumin seed (also called jeeraa) is an item used in preparing '*masaala*' (a mixture of food ingredient to add to the gravy). A method of preparation (Please see text box) was advised by a herbal doctor for a problem of digestion and general stomach ailments.

What is energization:

Energization is charging. If the molecules in the material lose electrons it becomes charged positively. If they acquire electrons then also they are charged but negatively. As explained earlier the charges that accumulate in a plastic comb is static charge. Same way certain materials rub with one another creates charges and also charges gets accumulated in them.

There are certain basic energizing methods followed in making herbal medicines. Grinding, heating, boiling, fermentation, and mixing with turbulence like water splash that creates negative ions in waterfalls are some of the methods that are usually followed. Even though an herb is referred to be used as medicine, the preparation is an important contributor in converting an herb to a medicine. Herb is an arrow. A tensioned arrow in the bow is the medicine. The arrow, which is having a static energy, would be dynamic when released from the bow and after releasing its energy it becomes static without any energy. Same happens from a herb to a medicine. Charge is imparted to the materials by the way we make the medicines. The charge in the medicine may gain the characteristic of the mixed products or only few. It is considered that the main herb plays a predominant part in the energized medicines. More analysis and research would help to advance in this area of dynamic materials.

Many ways to energize:

As explained in earlier chapter energized powders are made out of leaves, stems, barks and roots by drying the plant parts in the shade and then ground between stones or Mortar and pestle. Energized decoction is prepared by boiling the drugs in water. According to the hardness of the drug, multiple times of water is added to the drug and boiled to reduce till one fourth or one eighth remains. Sometimes various items are added, like oils, milk or honey. Energized paste is made from leaf, flower, bark, stem or root is ground by adding some water.

Infusion is a process of treating the classical herbs of tea leafs, mint, rose, jasmine and other flowers in water. The infusion is strained after the herbs are steeped for a few minutes. While steeping, the herbs should be covered. Hot infusion is by immersing the herbs in hot water for some time and cold infusion is the herbs soaked in cold water overnight. Sublimation is a process where the mouth of the bottle is kept open in the beginning and later closed to get the sulphur sublimated. Jam is a mixture of herbs cooked over fire stirring well and continuous until the recipe becomes semi-solid in consistency. Recipe should be taken out from the fire and allowed to cool and then mixing honey or some other already prepared herbal jams. This jam is called linctus and its storage pot preferred is porcelain. Trituration is the name of another method of processing materials to medicines. In one sense, it is a dilution of a potent drug powder with an inert diluted powder, usually lactose, in a definite proportion by weight. In another sense it is a form of reducing the particle size of a substance. The powders of herb and higher proportion of lactose would be ground and in multiple stages each time adding more lactose.

Some medicines are prepared by pouring a molten substance on a leaf. Another simple method is boiling the herbs in water until the preparation is reduced to one-fourth of the original amount like the cumin seed explained before. Some medicine systems use only one herb treated in boiling etc. to make a medicine. Uses of earthen pots were common and later on stainless steel utensils were used but never aluminium utensils.

Above are some of the methods prevalent in various places on earth. How the energy is imparted is only by treatment. The herbal persons resorted to these types of preparations when they did not get an improvement by raw medicines. Only the experience of handling various herbs in different ways taught these people. Various methods have evolved from their heads as thoughts and experiences and some are learned from neighbours and travellers from other regions. The valuation of their strength based on the content of energy is done only by few persons and some systems of medicine. One has to verify the medicines to find the energy added and to what extent.

Medicines to go into corners:

Simple herbs did not work and hence the old herbal doctors start the treatment of the herbs in different ways. To push the medicine deep into the inner core, modern medicine system makes most of the drugs with small molecules to make them penetrate the cell barriers. In pharmacology, organic compound of small molecule with a low molecular weight less than 900 Daltons is prepared. The idea is that this may help regulate a biological process, with a size on the order of nanometers (10^{-9}m). The small size has the possibility to rapidly diffuse across cell membranes so that they can reach intracellular sites of action.

Energy transfer:

Energy from one compound to another is like the elevated energy released in some form. This is similar to energy output in the form of light energy in fluorescent tube lamps. The electrons get elevated in gas atoms filled in the lamp and same electron falls to its original place releasing the energy. The energy released is in the spectrum of photons and we get light.

Different lamps Mercury or Sodium vapour lamps have different gases and outputs light with different colours. Light from sun is photon energy and this energy takes different forms later.

Energized medicines can travel crossing the barriers not as a material considered in modern medicine but as the effect of the material by way of charge it carries and the energy in it that helps the cure. In this way no material transfer is involved. When a compound is charged the energy levels of the electrons in the outer electronic structure get elevated. These charges stay until there is opportunity for its stabilization. The time the medicine is in the body there is a big commotion and lot of chances for the energy to be transferred or released. Same way as the electrons interact with molecules in a mercury or sodium vapor lamp to give out bright light, the medicine would output the energy in the body.

What is individualized medicine?

Dr. Rajan Sankaran of Mumbai, India classifies the people into three categories of what sort of medicine shall fit them. Any person's attitude and behavior will reflect his type and any of his health problems depends on his type, hailed from heredity. The three types belong to mineral, plant or animal kingdoms. For example a person has the attitude that he cannot fight back with others on any issues even if it is required when challenged for a fight and keeps quiet, belongs to mineral kingdom. One who gets provoked easily and is ready to hit back his opponent belongs to animal kingdom. The middle, who wants to fight but feels he is powerless, belongs to plant kingdom (Sankaran 2009).

The medicine has to fit the character of the patient and let us see a few examples for a clearer understanding. A person who walks in his sleep and does not remember the earlier night activity needs a medicine made from the parts of animal such as snake or nocturnal animals. Children eat all sorts of things not for fun, but due to the presence of some ingredient in those items that their system is in need. A kid, who craves for egg and not satisfied, may have problem in the calcium absorbing mechanism. Calcium salts which are contained in egg may be the medicine. In other words individuals craving will be the first indicator to understand on the selection of the medicine. Only experience could teach the physicians. If a medicine matches with the person then it would be the correct fix. This called balancing the disease and medicine.

In case the person's latest disease as found on the top of disease basket is cleared, the new symptoms that would surface next, will be different and the treatment would continue to clear the person's next problem. This would clear the disease basket one after another in a slow process. The relief in the first treatment would make the person to relax and confident that he is on the path to recovery. This course may take from months to years to clear all problems based on the person but a slow, steady and trouble free cure is what everybody desires. The patient should develop patience to stay the course for this process. Modern medicine is assuring and attracting the public that their medicine offers fast relief and cure. This image would eventually fade away only when individuals understand the progress in energy medicines and their safety and efficacy in their long-term benefits on health.

Energy levels:

Small charge in the medicine may help to handle surface problems. Slightly Higher charged medicine would help to clear somewhat deeper problems. Very high energy medicines would cross the barriers and make deep inroads into cells as there is only energy to transfer and not any material, which would find difficulty to cross barriers in the cells. Even mental and psychological problems can be treated when individual is treated as a distinct and unique entity than grouping by ethnicity, race, colour, region etc. In a sense, an individual is important and unique. Each one's constitution of body and mind is different from that of another and much like a finger print.

There are so many medicine systems around the world and showing their small presence in various communities as alternative treatment systems to modern medicines or with some name or even no name. There are many herbal treatments with medicines of energy and without energy. Some medicines induce the energy of the person to boost his disease fighting ability as activated system much like motivating a docile person. Few methods followed are supplying the energy itself as input into a person as if it is an energy boosting food.

It is more important to know
what sort of person has a disease
than to know
what sort of disease a person has.

-Hippocrates-

12

Energized medicine

Who has the power?

The messenger or the message?

The shooter, the gun, the gunpowder, the bullet
or
What the bullet carries?

You see the carrier
Can you see anything that is being carried?

Medicine shall be the carrier
to enter and to get out of system
in calm, quite and in peaceful manner
leaving behind
a
lasting cure.

Energy built in:

Our mind and body takes care most of our health problems and not the medicine. Medicines only aid them as a support to trigger the curing process and protect from outside disturbances. The bio systems get healed by their own internal processes. Our body has processes to treat the problems itself. Medicines do not heal. Medicines only help the bio systems for the cure. Same way others can only help and guide a person. If the outsider starts doing the main person's job then that person's system becomes lazy or weak, disturbed and gets deteriorated. Imagine the case of a person who starts doing a business. He can do only when he has interest. Others cannot do business for him. Others can only advice him and motivate him and that would help him to do business in an efficient and profitable way. Just handing over money cannot make him do business. The person should have at least some interest to do the business. He needs energy to thrive. Motivating the person helps him to do the jobs well. That is the energy for activation. Giving an investment with motivation for one to do business is akin to energized medicine for healing human body.

Many activities of mind by thoughts in an individual create a lot of biological changes and we consider this to be ailment of the body. A disappointment leads to frustration and that leads to resentment and anger. Anger increases the heart rate, arterial tension and more production of body chemicals like testosterone. It does not mean getting angry is bad. Even during his anger the body has to feel good and has to maintain the energy systems with good flow of energy properly. Venting his anger oneself is the best part of release, knowingly instead of uncontrolled. If the anger is not vented out, stagnation and energy blockages occur that eventually develop into disease. If anger continues, higher problem of rage and indifference starts. Overall activity in a mind starts secretion of some hormones and these hormones lead to some physical activity and these activities lead to generation of the production of some other chemicals. The wanting of oxygen, fresh air and certain vitamins in the body are pointed as reasons for a person to get angry. Many times fresh air is needed by the angry person apart from oxygen. The hidden truth is the requirement for negative ions present in air to aid in his mental energy. Instead of seeing the medicines looking inside the body, medicines should be analysed from the actions of mind, the origin of all ill effects in the body. The energized medicine plays a role here.

The mental changes make physical changes and the hormones act. Our body is made up of cells, which works on electric charges. A medicine carrying the energy enters into the body and inside the body the charges of medicine deals with the electricity and magnetic field. The old proverbs are "A thorn can be removed only by another thorn" and "you need a Diamond to cut a Diamond". These old generation sayings are valid as much today. The ionic charges only can deal with the electrically charged body.

There are many medicine systems and few have the energized medicines, some with calculated energy and other in a crude way but energized. When an industry makes medicines with all the measurements and the processes in calculated way the medicine's energy could be uniform and standardised.

A simple food prepared if chosen, taken and eaten with interest is the starting point of energy. Curiosity, interest and liking are foremost in food intake and digestion. When ground with saliva it adds energy and could be digestible easily. The energy, the food carries will resolve so many other issues of the body. Even with our advanced fast life if we match the speed of digestion and breathing system the energy would add automatically. Else our body cannot go along with natural life and we have to go for medicines.

Some of the important Systems which make energized Medicines are Ayurveda, Homeopathy, Bio-chemic Tissue Salts, Siddha, Unani, Chinese Herbal Medicine and so many other systems in practice widely.

Ayurveda (meaning Living knowledge):

Ayurvedic medicine is one of the oldest systems of healing that originated in ancient India. Ayurveda (Sanskrit word, aayur=life or living, and veda=knowledge) medicine utilizes diet, detoxification and purification techniques.

Ayurveda looks to how we can live in harmony with the greater universe. We disturb the balance when we ignore natural way of eating, eating food out of season, not following with internal requirements such as sleep and rest. When we disturb the balance between the inner and outer universe we become imbalanced. There are three basic concepts of characters (Doshas or humors) of the body are Vata (pronounced, Vaadhaa connected with air), Pitta (Pitthaa links with fire) and Kapha (kaphaa links with water) based on the idea that life force manifests as three different energies.

Vata supplies fuel (breathing, heart), Pittha works with the energy producing fire system (liver, bile, stomach). and Kapha regulates and cleans the systems (Kidney, urinary). Persons of Vata types are ruled by air and usually thin and angular, dry hair, strong, flexible and sensitive when in balance. Persons of Pitta types are ruled by fire and are typically with an athletic build, with broad shoulders and slim hips. When in balance, pittas have a strong mental focus and tend to be successful, decisive, courageous, and practical. Kapha types are ruled by earth and water and have a bigger build, thick hair, and when in balance, kaphas are stable, calm, patient, nurturing, and easygoing.

When thrown off balance, they can be lethargic, prone to depression, and overly attached. These three forces are present in everybody and are called metabolic types or constitutions. The balance of the three creates a good health and the imbalance is a disease.

Homeopathy:

Homeopathy is a form of energized medicine that arose in 1796 with efforts of Dr. Samuel Hahnemann of Germany. The bad experiences of the allopathic medicine, even at that time, as a doctor made him to search for alternatives and he ended up with a theory of 'Like cures Like' (In Latin *'similia similibus curentur'*). The energization process called potentisation of the medicines was his main philosophy. The doctrine of Homeopathy is when a substance that causes the symptoms of a disease in healthy people would cure similar symptoms in sick people. The concept of disease is that they are caused based on miasms, Psora (functional disturbances like skin etc), Syphilis (Deficiencies and ultra sensitiveness) and Psychosis (destruction like ulceration). The preparations of homeopathic medicines address these miasmic concepts (David Owen, 2007).

Homeopathic system can help from acute to chronic condition in ailment, but is the best for chronic illness and to clear the disease basket of any person. This is one of the medicine systems that could be utilised to improve the health of every individual preventing onset of any disease. The core theory of the constitutional nature of homeopathic medicines would help in this cause. It has been experimented that a single drop of homeopathic medicine of *'psoric'* nature at time of birth could help kids to be clear some basic problems and grow into healthy individuals.

Bio-chemic Tissue Salts:

Bio-chemic Tissue salts were prepared in the 1800s by a German doctor called Schuessler in the way of Homeopathy. The medicines that are made as tissue salts are only twelve. Schuessler found the reduction of certain salts in the body even in ppm (parts per million) level creates health problem in persons. The salts that have main importance in our system are Iron phosphate, calcium fluoride calcium phosphate, calcium sulphate, sodium chloride, sodium phosphate, sodium sulphate, magnesium phosphate, potassium chloride, potassium phosphate, potassium sulphate and silica. Potentised medicines are made from these naturally occurring salts. They are always mentioned in latin names (like kali mur for potassium chloride) also known as bio-chemic remedies or cell salts. Schuessler believed that a deficiency in one or more of these 12 salts led to disease in the body. He found taking any amount of salt did not increase the absorption after a certain level. He felt these salts would be absorbed more easily if potentised salts are taken. Potentisation is a form of energization (Schuessler, 1914).

These salt remedies are not supplements but weak homeopathic remedies. The amount of salt left in each remedy is too small for any nutritional benefit. As with all homeopathic remedies they are used only when symptoms are present and not repeated endlessly like food supplements. Tissue salts are limited in action compared to other homeopathic remedies. Due to low potencies they do not act deeply and not used for chronic diseases or mental symptoms.

Siddha (meaning extraordinary power):

The Siddha System of Medicine (Traditional Tamil System of medicine), which has been prevalent in the ancient Tamil speaking land. Like Ayurveda, Siddha is also a traditional medical system of India. It is of South Indian origin and has its entire literature in Tamil language. The basic concepts of the Siddha medicine are the same as those of Ayurveda. The difference is mostly in detail, preparation of medicines and treatment (NIS-Chennai, 2015).

The word Siddha denotes one who has achieved some extraordinary powers (siddhi). This achievement was related to the discipline of mind and its superiority over body, and was accomplished through both yoga and medicine. The medicine system was by persons called Siddhars and they made medicines by complicated methods even with certain compositions of compounds of mercury, sulphur, mica and several other metallic substances.

According to the Siddha medicine various psychological and physiological functions of the body are attributed to the combination of seven elements, first is plasma responsible for growth and development, second is blood and the nourishment imparting colour and improving intellect, the third is muscle, responsible for shape of the body, the fourth is fatty tissue, responsible for oil balance and lubricating joints, the fifth is bone, responsible for body structure, posture and movement, the sixth is nerve responsible for strength and the seventh is semen responsible for reproduction.

Siddha medicine also classifies the physiological components of the human beings as three humors, Vata (air), Pitha (fire) and Kapha (earth and water) like in Ayurveda system. When the normal equilibrium of three elements are disturbed, disease is caused. The factors, which affect this equilibrium, are environment, climatic conditions, diet, physical activities, and stress. In diagnosis, examination of subjects in test commonly known as 'eight tests' and these are tongue, colour, voice, eyes, touch, stool, urine and pulse. Out of all, the eighth, pulse reading is important.

The drugs used by the Siddhars could be classified into three groups herbal, inorganic substances and animal products for use as internal medicine and external medicine. There are many categories of preparations in Siddha medicine. The widespread preparations are decoction of plants, medicinal oil (thailam), electuary (laegiyam), and powder of dry herbs (chooranam). Many products with more complexity are not produced by all traditional practitioners because of the long time of preparation and the high cost of ingredients. Rare preparations are tablets and pills made of plants, minerals, metals, calcinations of minerals and metals, red powder obtained from preparations with metals, metallic salts and preparation of semi-solid based on mercury. Dosages are very small and diet (Called Patthiyam in local tongue) is strict in this system and some foods are forbidden during medication (Kandaswamy,1979).

Unani:

Unani (Yunaani Medicine meaning a medicine from Greek) is a form of traditional medicine is practiced in countries of the Middle East and South Asia. It has a tradition of Greek and Arabic medicine system based on the teachings of Greek physicians Hippocrates and Galen. The development as an elaborate medical system came in during Middle Ages by Arabian and Persian physicians, such as Rhazes (al-Razi), Avicenna (Ibn Sena) and Al-Zahrawi. Avicenna's 'The Canon of Medicine' has lot of influence over Unani. Even though Avicenna was influenced by Greek and Islamic medicine, he was also influenced by the Indian Ayurvedic medicine. Hence Unani had a major role in India from 12th century with establishment of Islamic rule over North India.

The concept of Unani medicine is based on the four powers or elemnents, the blood, phlegm, yellow bile and black bile in the human body. The theory of Unani suggests that these mixtures of four elements determine the temperament of a person. A predominance of blood gives a cheerful temperament; a predominance of phlegm makes one apathetic and the yellow and black bile make a person moody. Some doctors started following the concepts of Ayurveda using three characters of the body. In the diagnosis, clinical features such as signs, symptoms, laboratory features and temperament are important. After diagnosing the disease, principle of management of disease is determined on the basis of elimination of cause, normalization of powers and normalization of tissues/organs.

Chinese Herbal medicine:

Chinese herbal medicine is part of Traditional Chinese Medicine (TCM), which is a broad range of medicine practices sharing common concepts which have been developed in China and are based on a tradition of more than 2,000 years. 'Yellow Emperor's Inner Classic', a 4th century BC volume was the basis for the present day TCM. TCM holds that the body's vital energy (chi) that circulates through channels, called meridians, that have branches connected to bodily organs and functions.

All in the cosmos follows a certain pattern. The large celestial bodies like stars and planets are macro level and the elements of nature in those planets like earth in micro level. We are propelled by the same forces that are found in nature and follow the same process of cycles and patterns. According to the theories natural balance of Chinese, the earth has veins of energy that has paths through. There exists grids which are held together and all life derives its power. In the same all bio systems have the grids called meridians through which energy flows. These meridians are the energy grids and contain points on them that affect the meridians. These points are called acupuncture or acupressure points and are on the path meridians and are located in areas spread throughout the body from head to toe. Acupuncture points also have specific energetic functions depending on the meridian of specific organ. Other than herbal medicines acupuncture is one of the great systems which activate the energy system by passing on the energy through the meridians.

TCM is based on the observation of nature and we are nature manifested as living organisms. We, humans represent the juncture between the Cosmos and Earth. The concept of TCM is that what is good for one is good for other what is linked. What is good for the nature is good for humanity. What is good for the mind is good for the body. Harming one will affect the other and even harming part of the system would damage the whole. Harming one person harms so many others. The system is intermingled with one another. What is bad for the stomach is bad for the body. This philosophy does not exist in isolation and all mingled with one another.

The welfare as per TCM is a dynamic balance between these internal and external forces. Internal factors include the heredity, mind and body constitution, emotional, mental and spiritual aspects. The external forces are the climate, pathogenic factors, and the environment outside our body. Even a small imbalance in our body may cause a disturbance changing the harmony in the system. Unless corrected will lead eventually to a disease, which shows it a failure of our organism to go in harmony with the systems. The aim of the medicine systems of TCM is to help to maintain the harmony and create a balance between forces and assisting the individual to regain the level of normal person again.

The 'Five Element Theory', represented by wood, fire, earth, metal and water describes energy balances and correspondences within the body and outside the body and how these interact to generate health or disease and how do they regulate and are linked with one another. The theory provides a means of organizing and grouping concepts with five elements of nature and each relating to two parts of the body. Every element depends on the other element. Each element has control over the other element. Same way each part of the body controls the other parts and also depends on to the other parts of the body. Explanation in terms of elements would be clearly understood. With the base as earth it takes air and makes water and with that the tree or wood grows to give fire. Fire is the energy to the earth (Zhanwen Liu, 2001).

Linking the nature with body system goes from Earth for spleen and stomach, Metal (air) for lungs and large Intestine, Water for kidney and bladder, Wood for liver and gallbladder and Fire for heart and small intestine. With the base as Spleen and Stomach (earth) it takes the support of Lung and Large Intestine (metal-air) and makes the water systems Kidney and Bladder (water) and the food production with the Liver and Gallbladder (tree or wood) giving energy to Heart and Small Intestine (fire) to make the spleen and stomach work. That becomes a cycle. There is one creative cycle and another controlling cycle. Creative cycle is like Wood tends to create Fire, Fire tends to create Earth, Earth tends to create Metal, Metal tends to create Water and Water tends to create Wood. In controlling cycle Wood tends to control Earth, Earth tends to control Water, Water tends to control Fire, Fire tends to control Metal and Metal tends to control Wood.

The diagnosis depends on the eight patterns of Yin and Yang, Shortage and Excess, Interior and Exterior, Cold and Hot. For example the shortage may be with breathing. Also depends on the Six evil influences are Wind, winter Cold, summer Heat, Dampness, Dryness and Fire. Other subjects for diagnosis connected with the energy (Chi) used are Essence, Mind, Blood, Phlegm, Vital, Pathogenic, Stagnant, Stasis, and defiant.

TCM uses varieties medicinal plants. Some medicines are made combining more than eight to ten herbals. Chinese theory is based on yin-yang and defines the properties, Flavors, functional leaning and toxicity of the herbs. Every herb is linked with meridians and any of the five channels of the organs. Properties define the temperature characteristics of an herb such as cold, hot, warm, cool, and neutral. The idea is to prescribe a hot remedy for a cool problem. Flavors of an herb are sour, bitter, sweet, pungent, salty and bland. Flavors along with other characters decide a remedy. A sweet herb can remove the wetness of the body. Functional tendency is the rising and falling, floating and sinking of the herb. The functional tendency of the herb would correspond to the location of the disease with opposite tendency. Different substances may have different effects on the body meridians. Toxicity of the herbals are the another character of the herb and given such that the herb does not affect the body.

Combinations of two or more herbs make a formula. Some of the points considered in mixing are the compatibility, contraindication, and dosage. Combinations are made to have higher effect in its action and to reduce toxicity of the main herb. When two herbs are added the increase in toxicity is called incompatibility. Contra indication is an addition of another herb would reduce the effect of the primary substance and weaken. Preparations of herbs are in many ways. Decoction prepared in different ways with many combinations of medicines and multiple processes. Pills are made by combining the pounded fine powders of various herbs with highly viscous honey. Tonic is another from like a big honey pills. Powders are another form for easy absorption and are made adding granulated sugar or honey. Plasters are made adding powder mixed with wax of bees. Modern pharmaceutical technology created medicines of different forms such as tablets, tinctures, suppositories, capsules and drops.

Dieting here is not the amount or the calories but restriction on specific food items and is considered an important in Chinese herbal medicines. The diet system is sometimes like opposite such as the patient with cold symptoms should not take uncooked or cold food and of hot symptoms should avoid oily foods.

Dosage is decided based the combined action of the medicine and of extreme importance in the amount and the repetitions and depends on severe, acute, strong ailments, mild and chronic conditions, aged, frail, feeding mothers and children. Dosage is reduced as soon as the patient finds an improvement. Most of medicines are to be taken in empty stomach and food is taken only after one hour. Time of the day is important based on the medicines. Repetition is normally three times a day and for acute cases decoctions are prescribed once in four hours also (Jing-Nuan Wu, 2005).

Many others:

Many herbal medicines prepared with energy inducement. These are wide spread. Some village doctors make the medicine and they do not know anything about the energy but they know that the medicine cures. Such medicines shall be brought to the use of people encouraging the herbal doctors and helping them in making the medicines providing them with simple and clean facilities in a hygienic environment.

The medicine is the energy and not the food. Mixed food with varieties of grains, vegetables and fruits is the best food. Kids or any other person should not be forced to eat. Only the interest creation and inducement would make the food travel from top end to bottom end. Any food having allergy is very much connected with the medicine of his need. Only the best friend would be the worst enemy. Allergic item also has same characterisation. The food liked most by mind or body would become allergy. After the treatment the person would become normal in taking the same allergic food without any allergy.

Methods to establish cure:

Test methods for energized medicine cannot follow the allopathic system, the modern medicine. The medicine concept of small volume energized medicine is entirely different than the concept of high quantity modern medicines. Energized medicines shall be tested with people and not like the methods of modern medicine. Test should be on cure by individual methods of medicine and not copy and follow another method. Failures of modern medicines are due to their proving in animals. Due to the absence of chemicals, natural materials would leave the system once the job is done or not. The statistics of modern medicine should not be applied here. Same medicine for same ailment is not correct in modern medicine. One medicine may work for treating so many ailments. Many medicines may work for just one problem. Other simple treatments are available in energy medicine to activate the energy of a person.

The competent physician,
before he attempts to give medicine to the patient,
makes himself acquainted not only with the disease,
but also with the habits
and
constitution of the sick man.

-cicero-

13

Energy Activated to cure

When the man has energy
the messenger need not carry it.

But the energy within
to be
awakened
inspired
motivated
fuelled
kindled
stimulated
triggered
and
activated.

Sitting should get up to work:

When a person has serious illness in the body, the role of the medicine will be to correct the mechanisms and clear the toxins of the body. For an ailment in the body with its origin in the mind, thoughts or emotions, often times, the cure lies in tuning the mind, which would regulate the body. A person who lacks self-motivation or having reduced energy level needs some extra energy. The person's internal energy should be activated to get him into improved health.

A psychiatrist's talk motivates a person, stimulates and activates him. How? Where from the medicine is ingested into his system? Is there any medicine in material form really? If a person is not in a position to listen or think and react can the psychotherapist treat him? Psychiatrist is a person who analyses psychology whereas the one who treats is a psychotherapist. A person should have some basic energy level for the analyst to treat. Then comes the activation of energy, motivation of mind, driving his inspiration, encouraging his ideas, giving further impetus to his thoughts, stimulating his consciousness, promoting and comprehending the circumstances and creating an inner awareness. What do the lectures do? At least a therapist is in front of the person and interacts one to one, but not when hearing lectures. The first and foremost requirement is the person should have an interest within to listen. Then other actions will automatically follow. Lectures stimulate thoughts in a person and realize what actions one needs to do to achieve what his mind needs. The talk when imbibed stimulates thoughts in the mind, the actions follow and the life of the person changes taking a turn for his better. These mental strengths improve the physical status of the person giving him a fresh positive look at life and his future. A person, who feels unable to walk, walks initially on somebody's motivation and the little improvement seen by him boosts his confidence. This mental boost makes him walk further overcoming difficulties and soon he finds progress in days and the development changes his body to better and stronger. Here the mind and body benefit by mutual encouragement and synergy in thoughts and actions.

There are many treatments to activate the energy of the body

- Acupuncture
- Acupressure
- Yoga
- Bare foot walk
- and more such

Acupuncture:

The theory of Chinese medicine have same concept and is deep in the theory or analysis whether Yin-Yang concept, 'Chi' energy or 5-element theory. Traditional Chinese medicine theory in acupuncture is precise needling techniques, the principles of meridians, energy 'Chi', organ systems and safety methods. As per the theory, illness occurs when something blocks the energy flow or unbalances in the energy. Acupuncture is a way to unblock or influence 'chi'. Acupuncture is done by placing very thin needles into the skin at '*acupoints*' on the body. This is done to influence the energy flow through the needles. Acupuncture treatment is common in China, Japan and Korea even though differences exist between them in treatments.

During the visit of President Nixon to China in 1971, a New York Times reporter fell sick with appendicitis. The reporter cannot be brought to US because of the seriousness of the ailment. The American team was with the impression that the Chinese were following the age old methods and doubtful about the cure. No modern treatment systems like in US were found in Chinese hospitals during that time. However with no other way US authorities reluctantly agreed for treatment in

China. The surgeons in China successfully used acupuncture as anesthesia, during the reporter's surgery and subsequently to control post-operative pain. The ancient practice of acupuncture had come to the vicinity of western world with this event. From then acupuncture started spreading and people could get benefit out of it for many ailments.

Acupressure:

Acupressure is a form of touch therapy and is based on same principles of TCM. Acupressure is a therapy believed to have been developed before acupuncture and is the forerunner for the development of acupuncture. Acupressure acts shallow and acupuncture deep and very deep to the core. This therapy is considered as an important aspect of Asian treatment and mainly in Chinese medicine and Japanese treatments. Japanese acupressure is called Shiatsu. It uses precise points same as the acupuncture points, also called *'acupoints'*. These points follow specific channels, known as meridians or the same channels used in acupuncture pressure with finger over the points to activate the meridian path (Gala, 2003).

As per the legends Chinese observed some actions on the body of wounded soldiers during wars. Chinese healers studied the puncture wounds of the warriors and also some reactions on other parts of the body. Similarities among soldiers yielded certain interesting results connecting the affected part as stimulating point and the effect elsewhere in some other organs. Later by stimulating and observing the effects on the body the acupressure was developed as a treatment.

Acupressure is the non-invasive form of acupuncture. Finger pressure is used instead of the insertion of needles. This is one of the cost effective method of treatment and can be practised by self. Acupressure is used to relieve a variety of symptoms and also as a treatment for many health conditions, including headaches, pains, colds, arthritis, asthma, nervous problems, tension, sinus problems, sprains etc. Unlike acupuncture which requires a visit to a professional, acupressure can be performed by a layperson. Acupressure can be performed by a therapist or by a friend. What they need to know is the specific *acupoint*. Acupressure techniques are fairly easy to learn, and have been used to provide quick, cost-free, and effective relief from many symptoms. Acupressure points are stimulated to increase energy of the body. A better place of good natural air flow is recommended for more natural energy.

Yoga:

There are four basic forms in Yoga, the Breathing (Pranayama), Exercises (Aasanaas), Gestures (Mudhraas) and Meditation. The concepts are to earn more, spend well, spend less and save more. Each form may look different but they are under yoga and connected very much one to the other.

Breathing exercise (called Pranayama, meaning driving the life force) is to inhale more air, increasing of the air intake from the surroundings. The surroundings shall be with fresh air uncontaminated with the environment of trees, breeze as if air flow is controlled, good climatic conditions with fine temperature and humidity to concentrate more on the exercise than get diverted by disturbances. With pleasant music or background sounds and with all the above a relaxed situation occurs. Here what is talked is air and not just oxygen. The other ingredients of air are more important apart from oxygen. The breathing method not only enhances more air flow and also widens and cleans the paths of nostrils and windpipes. Lung plays a part in transferring energy in form of oxygen and ions to blood as a fuel. The *Praanayaama* increases the deep entry of air into the lungs and also increases the amount of air per breath and makes the lungs efficient. This is called earning energy from cosmos.

Exercises and Postures (*Aasanas* to pronounce *Aasanaas*, the postures). There are two types of *Aasanaas*, static and Dynamic.

Asanaas are to make the body active by circulating the oxygen throughout the cells. The static positions and dynamic actions create body movements so that the blood flow is channelled to all the parts. The exercise of *Asanaas* and their results can be observed only by experience after repeatedly practising them for some time.

> **Lungs - efficiency increase:**
>
> Air entry levels in the lungs are not deep and our short breath does not utilize the full capacity of the lungs. Normal efficiency is only 25% in taking oxygen and the lungs can go up to an efficiency of 70% maximum.
>
> Individuals who do breathing exercises and meditation reach an efficiency of 50%

Gestures (Mudras to pronounce *Mudhraas*, meaning mark or gesture) *Mudras* preserves the energy and make the energy circulated through the energy channels. The energy flow in our body is continuous all the time and the subconscious system tries to preserve it and our mind and physical external activity utilises it. All statues of Buddha will be depicted with a certain mudra. These mudras can be followed any time even when just sitting or in relaxation.

Meditation is a state to be practised to create a condition of mind for conserving energy. The thought process consumes more energy. A person with oscillating mind gets tired soon. A fast or strong decision maker (right or wrong) spends less energy and feels fresh than a person who struggles to decide and who tires fast. The meditation is concerned only with mind to develop the brain to consume less energy. The meditation is a practice to develop a concentrated mind. This practice would lead to a condition to have clear thinking, good concentration and mainly 'think one subject at a time' concept.

Meditation in the world is observed by different people in various ways. Just listening to somebody attentively, repeatedly writing the same word or sentence, uttering same words and sentences, reading a story etc. are some of the practices. In essence all are pointing to the need of mind concentration on one subject without oscillation and not thinking another subject until the one in the process is finished. Thinking of one or more subjects at a time but without oscillation is the need. This conserves body energy by reducing its input to the brain.

Bare foot walk:

Walking is considered important as an exercise because of limitations in available time and our fast paced life tuned to high earning, strenuous job, fast travel, quick-eating, short-nap, reduced sleeping hours and early wake-up to make the best out of 24 hours per day. With all this we are advised to do exercise like walking, yoga, tai chi, gym practice etc. To live the fast paced life we need more hours for this extra jobs else normal job may suffer. We do all the exercises in closed atmospheres and in limited spaces and the exposure to natural outdoor surroundings got reduced. Slowly only lately, the awareness is improving for outdoor activities such as walk in parks, gardening, supporting the planting of trees and sustain clean surroundings. Walking is recommended as the best method to lose the fat. Also it has been established that nature has provided us with acupressure points on the foot for the health of all vital organs in the body. We were designed by nature to walk on our bare feet for good health and only after embracing modern way of life we have started wearing shoes and live inside artificially air conditioned rooms.

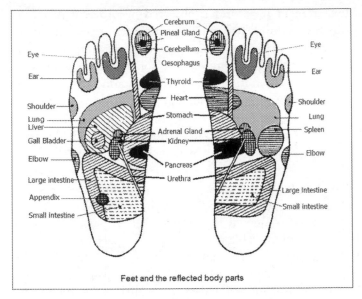

Feet and the reflected body parts

Fig-7

Natural walk is bare foot walk. Walking for few minutes with barefoot on soil makes the body to take some negative ions from the ground. The foot is not flat and the distances between the skin of foot and a flat earth would vary from point to point. Each point might have different pressure as it is supposed to activate a different organ of the body. The foot has been designed to have touch with the hard ground and stimulate the body parts to do actions. Let us utilise the design of foot by somebody and use it for our benefits. The feet, the hands and the ears have the links connected with all other parts of the body. The effect of a pin prick in certain part of the foot would get reflected in specific part of the body and hence is called Reflexology, the theory of which is used by acupressure. Fig.7 identifies the part of the foot and the other body part that it reflects. One of the simple and an easy method to good health is barefoot walk over sand five minutes a day.

More in our normal life:

Many of our action and the surroundings activate our energy without our noticing it or us even knowing about them. Also many methods exist to help activate our energy levels, like music therapy, psychotherapy, Silva method (Silva mind control) etc.

Music makes us relax and motivates many of us. A person on work with the background music concentrates on the work like a background of a picture portrays the basic picture with better visual appeal. A noise or disturbing music may spoil the person's work and concentration. The sweet music masks the disturbances and gives a soothing effect for the mind to be productive.

Psychotherapy is like somebody helping somebody else and in this case a therapist, specialised in the field of psychology does the job. A person who is not in a position to realise himself has to be made to understand. He should be advised what to do and how to do. A psychotherapist reads and listens to the person's problem, formulates a solution and makes the person realise and develop step by step as the mental activities take time for improvement. Here the energy of the person is tapped and awakened by the therapist and used to activate the person.

The Silva Method was created by Jose Silva in the 1950s and is a pioneer in mind empowerment research. With his observation and experimentation over his kids he dedicated his life to the awakening the minds of others. This method would put oneself into a relaxed frame of mind, and then using that relaxation for useful purposes like improving one's self-image, finding solutions to problems and increasing one's ability to accomplish goals. This method also develops students in getting better grades at school. The Silva Method is simple and straightforward. You simply close your eyes and take a deep breathing and go into a relaxed state of awareness called alpha state. When you relax, your brainwaves slow down and pulse at a certain frequency, known as "alpha brainwaves." The Silva Method is a away to use this relaxed state to accomplish things. After basic method Jose Silva came up with many deepening techniques. The Silva Method contains a host of other techniques, that you can use to solve your problems and helps you to accomplish your goals.

Much More:

Other than above so many other systems may be available around. They seem to appear as not of much value to us due to the non-propagation of them and lack of proper practitioners. Also the other dubious business oriented subjects occupy our mind in our everyday life and so we fail to notice them. Also some dubious persons misuse the energy systems for their profit and spoil the name. We have to search and find and use such good energy systems for positive living for our benefit. These are relaxing systems and the energy activation is a subtle process and not like medicines. Only the interest of the individual would help one to recognize and use the energy boosters. These techniques are mind boosters and in turn serve to bring improvement of the body.

The best doctor gives the least medicines.

-Benjamin Franklin-

14

Energy as Medicine

When the man has less energy,
charge with the energy

Then activate

Then medicate

Charging and regulating the energy:

We have seen the energized medicines and how they can improve our health. Also we saw few of the methods that can activate the energy in a person. There are simple methods to gain the natural energy directly through equipment even if we are not able to gain from the atmosphere. Also many healing therapies are practiced mainly based on regulating the energy of the persons.

Energy Treatments:

- Negative ion generator
- Pranic healing
- Touch healing

Negative ion generator:

Some scientists predict that future homes and offices will have heating and air conditioning systems that would produce and disperse negative ions. Until then, we can benefit from the revitalized and recharged environment by a trip to the mountains, seashores and gardens. We can also have the environment in our house enhanced with such energy giving gadgets in man-made ways.

Lack of negative ions is due to bad ventilation and reduced recirculation of outside air in air conditioning (HVAC) systems. Some air-conditioning systems have negative ion generation for filtering the dust from the rooms. It is recommended to have the ion generators to inject the negative ions in the ventilation system. Negative ions from the ionisers can improve health by reducing the dullness of mental activity and in turn tackle other minor ailments. Some of the ailments where the negative ions can help are mental instability, psychosis, mania, rage, clouded thinking, Depression, Asthma, Respiratory illness,

Dry hacking cough, Sinusitis, Arthritis symptoms, Joint pains and Nausea. They are very efficient air cleaners, particularly of the smaller sized particles. Ions can reduce the contaminants and pollutants such as dust, pollen, cigarette smoke and even vaporised substances like aerosol propellants and car fumes. Most ionizers will have a cleaning effect over a greater distance.

Caution is required in buying and using such gadgets. Humidifiers and vaporizers should not be used along with negative ion generators. Water molecules which absorb the negative ions are likely to form more positive ions. Unit shall be tested and proven and the ozone generation shall be within the permitted limits. Ozone is good in reduced volumes and not above the limits. Ozone is the best anti-oxidant and used to treat water to increase oxygenation. FDA of US specifies a limit of 50 parts per billion (ppb) of ozone in negative ion generators.

Negative ion generators are available to operate from home electric supplies, Car batteries and also computer's USB points. Negative ion generators work on the principle of "corona discharge", which is similar to lightning. A high voltage with a current limitation is applied to one or more needles produces ions. Electricity is a flow of individual electrons. And these electrons, supplied by the internal circuit, are passed to a needle towards the point due to high voltage. More negative ions repel each other and the ions are pushed out. By tuning the voltage level, designing the needle profile and materials this process is made very efficient to consume very less power. Table top generators plugged into mains supply are sufficient for common use. By the built in fan the negative ions are dispersed into the rooms.

Pranic healing:

The Healing by controlling the AURA is called Pranic healing (pronounced *'Praanic'* meaning life energy). Every bio organism has the electrical field of the body energy around it and that includes humans. Even a leaf removed from a plant retains the aura for some time. This aura can be photographed using Kirlian photography. The healer is trained to feel the aura of any person. The aura of a sick person would be irregular and that has to be tuned and that is the work of the healer. Once the irregularity is removed, the person's health would improve.

Pranic healing is a highly developed and experienced system of energy medicine developed by Grand Master ChoaKok Sui of Philippines. The prana or the cosmic energy maintains a state of good health. Fundamental principle is that the subtle energy from the atmosphere that surrounds the body has the power to energize the living entity and the body entity possesses the ability to heal itself and that the healing process is accelerated by increasing this life force. The healer increases the life energy and reduces the bad energy field.

There is a process for the removal of the bad aura. The healer never touches the person and handles only the aura. Hence pranic healing is called no-touch healing. The healer who regulates the aura around person's body should be healthy. The healer can draw in Pranic energy or cosmic energy from the surroundings. The healer is practised to feel the aura and he will remove the unwanted aura called the 'dirty prana'. The bad aura would be chopped by sweeping the hand. At the end of each sweep, the healer would flick his/her hands toward a bowl on the floor containing salt water. This salt water bowl would neutralize the dirty prana. The sweeping is done until the healer feels the patient's aura is smooth. The hand is normally one foot (30 cms) away from the person (ChoaKok Sui, 1990).

Touch healing:

People when they meet shake hands. Some who are close in family or friends embrace each other, Kids like to be touched, cajoled and played. Kids get energy from you without you and the kids knowing it. Hand is one of the tips of the body like leg and head where energy concentration is more. The hand to hand shake is not just physical. There is energy flow from one to the other and who has more automatically transfers to the other but in a mild way.

In American tribes the healer holds the hand of the sick and touches the head. This makes the energy from the healer to flow to the patient. In many treatments the touching is common. Some persons would not touch other under any circumstances and this practice has been developed for years with this idea of not losing energy. Touch makes energy flow from the healer. In some cases the energy of the sick is controlled like pranic healing. Touch Healing improves the health. It is not that the healer supplies energy in full to the other person. The small energy activates the person the way he is touched. The points that are touched are important like acupoints.

More Sources of Energy:

Many energy sources exist like light therapy, colour therapy, Reiki etc. In our normal life, we gain energy by various ways without ourselves even noticing it or knowing them. Let us also get the energy from the resources that we have lost contact with but still exist. Getting the cosmic energy through the negative ion generators is not that much a requirement when one could easily get same by good ventilation from outside air. A natural energy absorbed in the system through natural way would serve better purpose than an electrical device. Electrical devices can help the sick people like asthmatics as it produces large number of negative ions in one place. Always observe keenly the places that people show interest to visit and travel to. Hill stations, beaches, waterfalls, riversides, parks and gardens, house terraces, a walk among the trees and just a walk outside the house are important areas one thinks as refreshing or feels good.

Let us gain the information on all the energy medicine systems and methods practiced and utilise their benefits. Use the modern techniques to utilise the old sources, like using the modern technology of processing industries so that herbals can be converted into energized medicines. With the information technology and the analysing techniques that we have today, we can have the collection of data and dissemination of information about the characteristics of all the plants and herbals on the earth that can help the entire humanity in health.

"When all your energies are brought into harmony,
your body flourishes.

And when your body flourishes,
your soul has a soil in which it can blossom in the world.
These are the ultimate reasons for energy medicine—
to prepare the soil and
nurture the blossom."

Donna Eden, Energy Medicine-

15

Old and New

'Old is Gold'
is only in the saying now.
We want everything new.

We do not adjust to live in the land, in the soil,
in harmony with the plants, the animals and the space
that we have.

Below our feet the soil has limits but
overhead the space has no limit.
That is the reason man wants to reach out into space.

The time 'modern' started gaining control over the old,
the old lost all those skills gained over time.

The 'modern', which took over is only the loser
as it could not retain the skills.

Even now there is no new earth, no
new animals or no new plants.
The Base is old.
Only the Building is new.
We imagine as if we are in modern world

Our Nature was to self- learning but in modern times you are taught:

The modern society has improved our life using many of the old methods and practices, which have faded in our memory and some of those, were lost over time. When we encounter a problem with our so called modern advancements, we search for the old methods to tackle them, somewhat similar to our seeking out the help of the father, mother, old friends and relatives when we have a family dispute. Until such problems surface we live in comfort and one day when we search for solutions we may not be able to find them. That is the way the life goes. Human race, one to the other, started cultivating and teaching the habits to others making them think that they are intelligent and above all species. At the same time one started controlling other and ruling. By these ways of modern life, the individuals have lost their natural skills to acquire knowledge. Now, science is helping the human race to change the animals and plants such that they can also be controlled by humans.

Modern clothing and Natural cotton:

An example is the modern synthetics and the good old cotton clothes. After using synthetics for some time, we came to realise how comfortable a cotton dress is. We did not know that the use of synthetic materials all over the house absorbs all the life energy from the atmosphere in the room. Take the same example of asthma patient here and we attribute all the problems to cat, wool, pollens etc. All lead to the materials of ion absorption and reduction of negative ions in the air surrounding the asthmatic patient. Synthetic clothes and polyesters could absorb the negions as these materials are positively charged. Dress and bedding materials are to be carefully chosen for Asthma patients. Remember that the requirement of Negative ions is more for asthma patients than for a normal person. Especially the pillow covers and bedding shall be from natural material like cotton, else from synthetic materials with antistatic properties. Cotton clothes would help the patient to breathe all the normally available negions in the surrounding. One can notice that a Comb made by plastic gets charged when a comb runs through the hair. Same never happens with wooden comb. Synthetic dress adsorbs the negative ions of the air and ions that are required to be inhaled and adsorbed by the body get reduced. Cotton clothes are neutral and do not disturb the flow of negions. Use of cotton clothes would solve the problem if one is sensitive to the synthetics. Hypertension can be observed with persons who wear an excess of clothing especially when made of synthetic fabrics due to the reduction of adsorption of ions over the body.

Use modern and look at the old too:

Herbal and tribal medicines are being rooted out by modern medicines after benefitting from them to make modern medicines. After getting exhausted we could not find more herbs to cater to new diseases. One may think these are advancements. Any advancement, only when it is proven that it has helped the human race for generations

Famine – by simple transport in 1943:

Self sufficient methods in agriculture made the availability of food comfortable in Bengal state of India. When food became easily available from elsewhere the farmers of Indian Bengal state converted the paddy growing fields to grow jute. Jute was in demand to make sand bags required in war front.

One fine day the transportation system crumbled due to a calamity in the region of Burma, which was supplying rice. Japanese occupation of Burma made it so. In other parts of India all the transports were carrying military aids and sudden diversion of transport was not easy to supply food from elsewhere. Farmers could not start their rice production due to seasons and time needed to change crops. Famine started in weeks and the result is death of around 3 million people.

has the right to qualify. Any short term development in science may not prove its use. Once the same science destroyed the basic foundations easily the systems that existed for millennia would be decimated. Whereas the short term science has been seen to fail and even reverse its own findings within just few decades. Science has advanced the facilities for the comfort of human society but has not enhanced in quality. Careless developments in agriculture have created famines one century ago (See the text box).

Science eliminated by this advancement many of the old basic man made systems. Horse cart and bullock carts were replaced by automobiles and fertilisers replaced the natural manure in use till then. Natural oil lamps and candles replaced by electricity and wood burnt ovens replaced by gas cookers. All the new methods improved our living and we discarded the old methods and systems to embrace new technology. Then the time has come that we cannot utilise the automobiles due to fossil fuel shortage and its unavailability due to high cost. Now, the high cost of transport from place of manufacture to the market where it is in demand tends to hinder the mobility of people. It is not that we have to ride bullock cart, but to know that the need of the old would arise and by that time we would know nothing to cling on to.

After the advancement of computers we started storing all information in the new media. The media in which we were storing information changed from paper that existed for centuries, to computers and DVDs at present. Basic advice is to forego the books and print on paper and all information should be in digital format and virtual books as eco friendly. Why do we have to throw the paper books from homes and offices with the reason that we have got the computers? Let books remain alongside with computers. The storage of information in computers never got stabilised even in last ten years and we are being advised to change to digital format. Once converted to digital, the old books and the palm leaf manuscripts are thrown to a corner and are lost forever. Many books and research of recent times exist only in virtual format and its fate would be known when we could not access. We never realised that the old palm leafs and the books are the information on which we lived once. The same old information from books is going to help us if we preserve them. Else, we do not know when the computer media stabilisation is going to take place- perhaps it would never will! Starting with 5¼" floppy discs to 3½" floppies of single density, double density and high density and to CDs and then to DVDs of single layer and double layer and we are now in portable drives called USBs within past 50 years. In comparison, just imagine the fact that papers lasted us for centuries being eliminated in just few decades! Papers need only our normal eyes to read under natural light anywhere unaided, where as the computer media needs power source, much hardware and a hidden computer program to be relied upon to perform in-between.

Present technological advances have the requirement in volumes of data and information. The value of that data is not considered and volume is given importance because of the capability for the high capacity storage we developed. Where do they store and in what form? Volumes of documents written two thousand years back remain even now worldwide in many languages. Is it possible with modern media to stay through centuries? What happened to the data stored in the floppies 30 years back? What about the program that read it? What about the computer that had the program? Program is changing and the computers too are changing and media changing faster than computers. All are in virtual forms and one day would become virtual by the same technology that produced it and may stay in memory for a generation and fade away in the next. If that history remained written in books we may be able to read and bring the advancements from back to front when needed. This is same case as music disks to audio tape rolls to audio cassettes and now all in the virtual media.

If no transport is available, one can still walk or take the bicycle, which would probably remain, but not the knowledge base, the book. One needs external electric power from morning until midnight and even while sleeping, for 24 hours. We need energy for anything and everything. We did not have the electric power few centuries back and our forefathers were living for millenniums without it. Why this turmoil just in the last 100 years? Let us live modern lives and let the old remain alongside with us- for we do not know when it would be needed again?

The trouble with modern society is that it makes everybody go behind something without knowing what is leading them in front. As long as it is attractive and helping our life it is fine. We think we are intelligent and we can write the volumes of teaching materials, develop teaching methods, guide books and train the teachers to educate the kids. The hard fact of the reality is we are limited in our knowledge than our forefathers. Our forefathers allowed us to learn. Just few years back, anybody can do research and they did and invented a lot because of the freedom of their thoughts. But now the freedom is within the boundaries of laws, rules and procedures. The new inventions are often only sub set of the old. Even with all the advancement in science, we do not have tools to measure the five basic senses and not even the daily problem of pain with everybody. The reason may be that we have not invented the method to measure and no units to compare and evaluate.

Senses and science:

Nature provided us the senses to find food and eat. What the animals have now is the same as what we had and what we still have. Animals used them before and continue to use even now. We used them before but we forgot how to use them now. We think we know more than what the animals know. But we have been losing the acuity and sharpness of our senses over time in the past few centuries and at even faster pace in the last few decades. The animals are still using the senses of seeing, smelling, tasting, hearing and touching but we are not utilising these senses in the same way as we did years back.

We had all the senses to find food, eat and survive. We were searching for food like animals. The laziness to search for food made us to collect and store the food and eat at our convenience. When only a few persons went to collect food for others, we lost the senses of touch and feel of the items and smells to identify the right tasty food. The taste of cooking changed the natural taste we had for food. Again the laziness to go over distances in search of food paved way to start agriculture and produce food in one place and encouraged us to sit and wait for food to come to the table. By reduction in number of farmers, the cultivators of food, the technology started to feed us the food from the processing industries than fresh from the farms. The basic underlying motive to all this is to make someone lazy if you want to gain and exercise control over him.

We use the same senses even now for watching entertainments and the colours of food supplements on television, to enjoy the smell of artificial flavours, to eat based on the industry's advertisements, eating more and dieting more, travel in cars and then do exercise in gyms. If we live a healthy and happy life nothing is wrong with such modern life style. By technology whatever has been developed, with its measurement and units, using mathematics has been widely put to use for the benefits of technology like electricity, mechanisms, communications, chemicals, nuclear technology etc. They are widely accepted by the population. We are able to measure length, weight, electricity, light, magnetism, charge of an electron, atomic weights etc. and even thickness of human hair and molecules up to nanometre level. All these technical fields have input of units and calculations. Even though biological sciences have grown, no unit is developed for the five senses of our body basics. Science and technology progressed wherever it entered with a reference and to measure further. Every physical entity can be measured with its units and measurements. If at all we want to utilise our senses, the five senses shall have unit of measurement with a basis of mathematics and exploiting the known laws of physics, chemistry, engineering and technology. We have not been able to evaluate so far the measurements of these senses. Hence the senses did not improve in us and we lost what little we had in the previous few centuries. We cannot measure the smell, taste, feel of pain and look.

How did we use our senses to eat? Eating starts with seeing the food at first. When you see a fruit or a vegetable you know that these are things you can eat and good for your health. The shape and colour attracts you to pluck it from the tree. The smell also attracts you to put it to your nose even subconsciously. Sometimes you see and take in your hand and feel it. The feel makes a sense to reject or accept it. The skin of the fruit may itch or be greasy and one's affinity to it depends on the person too. Once you like the fruit, you may want to pinch and taste a bit of it. A good taste in your mouth makes you eat more. When you start eating, the way the fruit makes a sound in your mouth increases the interest or wants to reject. The sound depends on the grip with the teeth and in its biting or munching. Animals continue to do their eating with the senses they have, the same old senses they have retained. How about us humans? Do we need the senses back to natural form from artificial form is the question? One example of losing a sense is nowadays we never bite an apple which improved the strength of teeth and massaged the gums and instead we make apple juice so that the teeth take rest.

If we could get back our senses, we can select the modern industry food, feel it, smell it, taste it and eat it and easily decide its quality too. We would recognize easily and reject the artificial smells and tastes. We would be able to differentiate between the good and the decayed and the rotten. We do not have any instrument to measure the smell of rotten. The range of smells is supposed to extend from the sweetest smell to rotten smell. In absence of this type of instrument to measure smells we find the bad food by inference from type of bacteria in the food to tell us if it is good or bad.

We need not go back to find the paleolithic food of a bygone era. The progress of technological advancements is mostly in the mechanical sense and in the way we perceive life. The science should help develop the life sciences, in real sense not just for records. Only then we can utilise the resources of nature.

Root out the roots of plants:

The human society and mainly the modern society, that we live in the developed and developing countries, has embraced artificial comfort neglecting the natural environment. By this, the human race has alienated and moved away from nature and natural surroundings by cutting trees, spraying herbicides, modifying the plants genetically, tampering with nature for fast and short growth. After carrying out large scale destruction of nature, we start preaching about felling trees and green movement. Nature can and will endure unlike manmade structures. Once the artificial life gets degraded, the people will start realising the value of living in harmony with nature, the nature that was already spoilt by mankind in the name of modern technology. GM (Genetically Modified) product is like growing a plant in a controlled environment. With the genes modified scientists may not know how the growth will be in its natural climatic conditions, including the requirements of water, manure, temperature, humidity etc. This would take years to prove and need many generations of plants and humans. This is like growing an animal in its artificial environment like zoo than leaving it to roam in the forest in its own natural surroundings.

How to design for a healthy life:

Information - Making the most of nature's potential using modern science should be the target. The same time we have to preserve the past history, old documents, remember the findings of old scientists in a simple way that would lost for long. Apart from teaching science, our kids should be made to learn the nature, understand the nature. Create the situations where they know how to live and how to use their knowledge. Make them learn on their own. Do not teach and thrust information onto them.

Homes - Some people have even suggested that if staying inside a pyramid is so healthy, maybe we should redesign some of our buildings to be in that shape. Some people believe the patients would recover more quickly in pyramid-shaped hospitals. Children would learn more quickly and easily in pyramid-shaped schools. Families in general would live happier, healthier and congenial lives in pyramid-shaped homes. Utilise the modern solar panels to tap the energy of the sun. We need studies that are focussed more on the benefits to human health than for more benefits to the industry on effects of electromagnetic frequencies from high voltage electrical transmission lines, mobiles etc.

Dependency - Plants need the nature, soil, rain, wind etc. and not animals or human race. Animals need plants and soil and not human race. Human race needs animals, plants and the nature. We need all to sustain our lives.

Skills - Industries never cared for the human skills and converted them as skills of machines. Human skills took hundreds of years to develop and machine skills in decades. What is the future should there be a cut in the link? No skills would be available in neither machines nor men.

Feed - We grow chicken in an artificial way to be consumed and we do not eat the natural chicks that grow in nature, because of the need of huge quantities commercially. At the same time, we feed more grains to the cattle and chicks to get more meat. The grains that we feed to the cattle would be sufficient to feed all the people on this earth.

Health - Manufacture good quality ion generators using the modern facilities and the technology. At the same time tap from the environment that provides us with cosmic energy from nature. Utilise the modern processing to manufacture energized medicines. Every medicine system shall use the herbs of that locality based on the botanical species. Even though other similar medicines may work, the herbs around the habitation of concerned population would be more compatible.

Where there is UP there would be DOWN:

There are so many treatments for the improvement of heath. What is talked as medicines as energized, energy activated are only few. So many other treatments through energy, by energy and energized medicines may be available. Only the individual's interest would find the best suited for him amongst the wide spread variety of treatments available.

Whenever we advance and gain something for future we are losing something of the past. When we climb the ladders we think we will not have to return and kick the ladders away. We never look back to see what we left behind. By this way, we have only left a spoilt legacy for our future generations. We never felt the importance of natural ways that have sustained us over the past several generations for centuries and we seek to discard them without realisation that one day they will come in handy when we fall or forced to climb down due to human folly in pursuing a wrong path. We only think both will not happen.

"Learn from yesterday,
live for today,
hope for tomorrow.
The important thing is to
not stop questioning."

-Albert Einstein-

16

Future

Let us all
live in peace with the surroundings
with the people around
with the animals, birds and plants
with this earth and with mother nature

If we do not like something
let us stay away
but let us
not ruin or decimate

We are enjoying many energy forms without our knowledge.
Some may be in destruction
If we know what they are
we can utilise them
better and
preserve them
for the coming generations

Future is always bright. Else we will not move forward:

Life is a one way path. We cannot return back. Old useful and useless go out and new useless and useful come in. We are struggling to decide whether the new advancements in science and technology and mainly in medical field are useful or not. More than a hundred years ago we were using many herbal medicines. After a great cycle of evolution of modern medicine and its advancements, we have realised it as an illusion and now we are searching for older treatments of any form to get a cure. We do not say that only herbal medicines in energized form are a cure for all. Many more may exist. This trend would continue and change the requirement of new types of medicines. The allopathic medicine would take some other form as it cannot cater to the need of people who face new diseases and threats from new viruses. People are losing confidence in the allopathic medicines, due to its inability to cure and being faced with new health problems and side effects due to consumption of more drugs than food items.

Medicine systems and Medical treatment:

Many believe medical treatment is science. It belongs to category of mathematical statistics as applied to nature. Medicine uses mathematics, physics and chemistry and not medical treatment. Just to create public interest the industrial and business society adds every subject on earth to science like political science, environmental science, biological science and even natural sciences. Political science cannot predict who will win in an election. They need to conduct a survey and decide with a probability factor adding some allowances. Environmental science cannot predict when will be the next cyclone or earthquake or even rain. All are expected or likely events. Biological science and natural sciences can work with statistics as a bridge with judgements, likelihood, chances, possibilities, probability etc. Hence medical treatment is not science. If it is science we should have improved our health of the whole generation of people.

All the treatments and cure are based on chances. Each medicine system has its own method of treatment. The chance of cure is more important and it is statistics, like 'few out of many' got cured. Each system has advantages and disadvantages. One system may not treat all diseases. The idea should be that patient shall be cured, whatever the system of treatment may be. Cure should be the important requirement. But many doctors consider that their system should be the followed like a religion. Also cure shall be the goal and not mere suppression of the symptoms. The energized medicines could work for cure. Medicine highly energized can travel to the level of cell in the brain. Such medicines go to the source of the problem and not only to the part that is affected. With the advancement of medicines, the disease causing germs have developed resistance. The non-availability of medicines for new diseases made people to search for new avenues where they could get salvation from health troubles. The World Health Organization (WHO) estimates that 80 percent of the population of some Asian and African countries presently use herbal medicine for some aspect of primary health care.

Allopathy to other medicines:

Statistics shows nearly one-third of American citizens switch to use of herbs for a cure. Unfortunately, a study in the New England Journal of Medicine found that nearly 70% of people taking herbal medicines (most of them were well educated and had a higher-than-average income) were reluctant to tell their doctors that they used complementary and alternative medicine. (UMM-University of Maryland Medical Center). NCHS (National Center for Health Statistics) of US in a survey in 2007 lists the number of people who go to alternate medicine systems. 11.8% of children (below 18 years) and 38.3% of adults use alternative medicines. The persons who used the energized medicines such as Ayurveda, Acupuncture and Homeopathy are 1.6% of children and 3.3% of adults of the American population (American Health, 2010).

Future systems for cure:

We should be clear why allopathy medicine cannot be fit for health. As a medicine they are synthetic or extracted chemicals and not natural. Our body can adjust only to naturally available materials. They are not active materials for action with a force to cure. Only energized materials could work in our body as medicine. Non-energized would stay in the body and do something contrary to nature. Energized medicines can cross any barriers in the body due the energy transfer. Allopathic medicines are manufactured so that they can cross the cell barriers. Most of the medicines are small molecules and less than 500 Daltons. Even skins cannot absorb molecules heavier than 500 Daltons. Medicine as material cannot cross many barriers where as the charges can (Bos JD, 2000).

Allopathy medicine assumes any growth in the body should be operated. The growth is due to some problem of the biological system and not by any external actions. In that case body biology should be able to solve the problem by way of the medicines.

Many of the tests are in gross scale and not what is in the body. For example in biochemistry tests are done for minerals like sodium, potassium, calcium etc. What is present in the body is not sodium or calcium or phosphorus but different type of mineral salts like sodium phosphate etc. Based on the rough value of minerals its supplements are prescribed. That is the reason for mismatch between the requirement and the supply.

The prescriptions are based on tests of body contents and body scanners. The present instruments and equipment can measure only up to certain accuracy. Day by day the technology is developing equipment to a better accuracy but many of the observations have a limit. The major parameter, pain, is yet to get a good instrument. In view of the system not being able to cure, many cures have been renamed as management like pain management, cancer management etc.

Testing of medicines with animals and testing medicines based on diseases cannot equate to other systems of medicine. With the lack of knowledge of other systems of medicines comparing them with modern medicines have no value.

Even though there are many systems of energized medicines that can be adapted for use, certain medicine systems have been well developed for centuries and also well proven. At the same time all the systems of energy medicines need to be developed and optimised for its effect for the ailments. In view of the degradation of allopathy system of medicine, the alternative systems that would find favour with the people are Acupuncture, Ayurveda and Homeopathy. Allopathy would be the system mainly for surgical operations needing urgent intervention and correction. The two energized medicine systems, Acupuncture and Ayurveda crossed many centuries in proving their effectiveness and now are spreading to other places from the place of their origin. Homeopathy, even though it served for 200 years, has proved its usefulness still it is called as placebo by some. People who have no knowledge of this system cannot pass judgement on the effects of this energy medicine. For improving the health, the body does not know religion, race, colour, ethnicity, country, origin or anything. The public should follow the treatment where they can get cure for their problems irrespective of the medicine systems.

Acupuncture would be the choice for general treatment. Starting from acute to chronic problems best system is acupuncture and this system is widely used and has proved its effectiveness. Many physicians use acupuncture and Homeopathy at the same time.

As part of TCM, the Traditional Chinese Medicine, acupuncture and acupressure play a major role in treatment. Acupuncture treatment is through an energy layer just below the skin. Acupuncture system involves the use of sharp, thin needles, which are inserted in the body at very specific points. These points are called '*acupoints*' or acupuncture points and are traceable in the path of meridians of the basic file elements of TCM. This process helps to remove the unbalance in the system and is used to treat a wide variety of illnesses and health conditions.

The history of the acupuncture dates back to 5th century BC. Stone needles were in use in that era. Nowadays needles made of stainless steel, copper and silver are in common use. The concept of five element theory and yin-yang is applicable to acupuncture also. The energy called Chi plays a vital role in the treatment. As per the Chinese theory the energy Chi is the fundamental life energy of the universe. It is in the environment and invisible. We inherited the energy from birth and we get the energy from air, water, food and sun. The energy for healing is imbibed thru the needle when it connects the atmosphere and the energy layer. This is the energy in atmosphere called the cosmic energy prevailing everywhere in space.

The energy travels through the path of meridians of the twelve main organs connected with the five elements earth, metal, water, wood and fire. The twelve main organs are the lungs, large intestine, stomach, spleen, heart, small intestine, urinary bladder, kidney, liver, gallbladder, pericardium, and the "triple warmer", which represents the entire torso region. Each organ has its own energy connected with it and interacts with particular emotions or the mental states. Chinese doctors connect symptoms of the patients to their organs. Each acupuncture point in the meridian of that particular organ has significance in selecting it for treatment. One or more acupuncture points are chosen to insert the needles for the treatment.

The organs and elements are related to physical and mental symptoms. Problem of one organ has an effect over the other also. The links are complicated but the Chinese medicine system has established the connection between any two organs, and the disease is seen as an imbalance in the meridians of the organs. Balancing the energy by establishing its intrinsic harmony between the organs by passing the chi, the energy through needles is the goal and the treatment helps to bring back to normal health.

Disease can be caused by internal factors like emotions, stress, anxiety and tension and external factors like the environment and weather, and other factors like injuries, ordeals, diet, and germs. The infection is not considered as a problem due to germs and viruses, but primarily as a weakness in the energy of the body. Two sicknesses are never the same as per the system and each person's body has its own characteristics of symptoms, balance and imbalance. Acupuncture is used to open the path and adjust the flow of the energy 'chi' throughout the organs (Longe, 2002).

In humans the cosmic energy is obtained from the air by the acupuncture points and distributed throughout the body. The points are small regions on the body surface to a size of approximately 1mm in diameter. In Moxibustion treatment dried mugwort (a small spongy herb) is burnt near the needle to generate fumes that increase ionic charges of both types, negative and positively charged molecules. The ionic charges of negative type can reach the needles due to its freedom compared to the positively charged heavy molecules. This way the energy reaches the needles that will enter into the meridians. Moxibustion is used only when the patient has deep health problem like a chronic disease that requires high chi energy. The selections of right time in a day for treatment are considered important based on the presence of high energy in the atmosphere (Claudia Focks, 2008).

Homeopathy was created, as an alternative to modern medicine, in 1796, by Samuel Hahnemann based on his doctrine of 'like cures like'. Homeopathy was very much popular in the 19th century due to the bad treatment in cures existed at that time. Hans Birch Gram, a student of Hahnemann, introduced the system in the United States in 1825. In 1835 first homeopathic school was opened. Many homeopathic institutions appeared in Europe and the United States throughout during the 19th century. There were 22 homeopathic colleges and 15,000 practitioners in the United States in 1990. Main reason for the success of homeopathy was its effectiveness in treating people suffering from infectious diseases and during epidemics. During epidemics, diseases such as cholera, death rates in homeopathic treatment were very less compared to allopathic treatment. Many allopathic doctors had interest in homeopathy and started practicing and were famous by their practice.

Homeopathy was prevalent in US during the formation of American Medical Association (AMA). Two persons were important in running the AMA dictatorially from 1899 for half a century. George H. Simmons and Morris Fishbein both served as general manager of the organization and as editor of its journal JAMA (Journal of AMA) and were called "medical Mussolinis.". AMA was a weak organization with little funds. The advertisements in the medical journal started the revenue and Simmons planned to transform the AMA into a business organisation. The drug companies were made to get approval of AMA called "seal of approval" and were forced to advertise in JAMA and its various affiliate publications. Homeopathy slowly disappeared leaving a few traces with the rise of AMA and the allopathic drug companies with AMA's support (Ullman, 2007).

The homeopathy continued in eastern countries where some homeopaths continued to practice irrespective of the progress of modern medicines. Even though the practices continued in Germany, France and other European countries, the revival was mainly due to a Greek homeopath George Vithoulkas in 1970's. The use homeopathic medicines in US and Europe are increasing year by year (Vithoulkas, 2002).

Homeopathic medicines are named with basic Latin names such as Belladonna, Nux vomica or Alumina, CalcareaPhosphoricum (calcium phosphate) etc. Numbers of remedies are more than thousand and increasing based on new requirements.

The medicine is in energized form or called potentised form made from one herb. What is this process called potentisation? Homeopathy follows a method to energize a material either a mineral or plant or an animal product. Also diseases products and allopathic medicines like paracetamol are converted to energized forms. Potentisation is also called dynamisation using the processes called 'Succussion' and 'Trituration' (Lockie, 2006).

Succussions is a method where the drugs that are soluble in Alcohol or Water are diluted serially in stages with the media either alcohol or water and every dilution is followed by vigorous jerks and impacts of the liquid solutions. This makes the solution as the collusion of water particles and gets energized. Trituration is similar to succession but for the drugs that are not soluble in liquid media using lactose, Sugar of milk, instead of liquid. The dilutions are done mainly on 'Decimal scale' and 'Centesimal scale' using the media. The media like Alcohol, Water, and Lactose are called as carriers or vehicles. In decimal scale the dilutions and triturations are prepared in the proportion of one part of the medicine to nine parts of the media. In decimal the original drug substance will be one part and media 10 parts. After energizing one part from eleven parts will be taken and fresh 10 parts of media will be added and again energized. If done 6 times the potency is called 6X and X represents ten. Same way centesimal is done with dilution of 100. Here 30C means diluted and potentised 30 times and 'C' represents 100. Increase of potency reduces the content of basic material but

> **Avagadro number:**
>
> The explanation below is to show that the homeopathy medicine may not have even one molecule of the herb in it when the potency crosses 24X or 12C. That means material may not exist. One can imagine in higher potencies like 1000C what would be the material. The energy is the impact crossing all barriers of the body.
>
> Assume carbon (graphite) is the medicine and 12 grams of carbon would have $6.2x10^{23}$ molecules. The value $6.2x10^{23}$ is called the Avagadro number. 1 gram of carbon would contain around $5x1022$ molecules. How many molecules one can expect in a medicine of potency 24X? The chance or the probability even for the presence of one molecule is very less.

increases the charge to a higher level. Doctors who are not aware of the energized medicine call these medicines as equal to the effect placebo, a dummy. Homeopathic remedies are prepared in numerous potencies that can manage deep-seated chronic problems as well as simple complaints. The effect of medicine on the sick will be slow but steady and not fast as the allopathic, which creates turbulences during the action of the drug.

In homeopathic treatment primary importance is given to mind and then parts of the body. After selecting the homoeopathic medicine by the process of comparison of the drug picture with disease picture of the patient, the medicine is chosen. Normally a single remedy would be prescribed taking all the symptoms into account.

Ayurveda has established its usefulness for centuries and commonly used for acute to chronic problems. Ayurveda is considered one of the best medicine systems useful in physiotherapy. The theory of Ayurveda treatment is to balance the three elements or the forces or the vital energies Vata, Pitta and Kapha. The imbalance is considered as a disease. Every one of us has some portion of these three elements. These elements decide our mind and body constitution and whichever force is high that dominates our movement, transformation or structure. Vata person is inclined to be thin, light, enthusiastic, energetic, and changeable. Pitta tends to be intense, intelligent, and goal-oriented. Kapha is an easy-going, methodical, and nurturing (Chopra, 1990).

The basic principle behind ayurveda is "like increases like." So to maintain energy and balance, you need to gravitate toward the elements unlike those inherent in your constitution. Since you already have those qualities in excess, reducing them can help you find balance. An example is a vata person, doing a vata activity, in a vata season would increase vata. A better way for a vata is be to bring in more elements of pitta and kapha.

Famous texts on medicine and surgery on Ayurveda are Charaka Samhita and Sushruta Samhita. The Sushruta describe 125 surgical instruments, 300 surgical procedures and classifies human surgery in 8 categories. The Ayurvedic classics mention eight branches of medicine. The form of products in Ayurvedic medicine system are Juice, Powder, Decoction, Paste, Hot Infusion, Cold Infusion, Medicated Oil and Ghee, alcoholic Preparations, Pills or Tablets, Scale Preparations, and Collyrium etc. Many oily preparations are for physical problems like rheumatism, joint pains, muscle restrictions etc.

Ayurveda has eight ways to diagnose illness, called pulse, urine, stool, tongue, speech, touch, vision, and appearance. Ayurvedic practitioners approach diagnosis by using the five senses. Initial examination of a patient consists of observation, touch and questions. Observation is to evaluate general physical health by look, the person's movements, body structure, skin and eyes, facial lines, nose, tongue, lips, hair, and nails. By touching the patient, Ayurvedic practitioner checks the palpitation. Then questioning is to listen to complaints, symptoms and to listen to the mental and psychological conditions. The exhaustive examination helps the Ayurvedic practitioner not only diagnose the disorder, but individualize or tailor treatments for each patient. The individual is supposed to have the basic energy to bring the body back to a healthy and balanced state.

The treatment would be decided not to look at healing the illness, but to concentrate on the methods that would strengthen the basic three elements inherent in every body. In turn the individual would recover to health. The process in Ayurvedic system is to help the body to make its own energy to heal. Treatments and medicines would act to support the body's mechanisms in its self rejuvenating process. Other treatments include massage, breathing exercises and physical treatments. Physical treatments are the specials in Ayurveda. Panchakarma (five actions) is one consisting of five therapies to detoxify the body and balance the three elements. Another technique involves dripping of medicated oil on the forehead.

Patient would be prescribed with herbal medicine in the form of liquid mixture treated with oils, pellets, tablets and powders. Dietary instructions are tailored to each individual's constitution, with the six primary tastes in mind. The patient is supposed to follow dietary instructions and mainly what not to eat during medication. Normally medicines are to be taken in empty stomach with a gap of at least an hour before and after food.

Energized treatments:

Above three systems have similar concepts in medicine considering the mind and body as part of a person. 'One patient one physician' system is followed in these treatments. All diseases are connected with one person. One disease creates many symptoms. Every symptom of one person is analysed and he is the physician. The physician shall be one to take care of the sick individual to clear his disease and make the person healthy. These medicine systems are simple and cost effective.

Allopathy, the modern medicine system, out of all medicines, would be the system primarily for surgery. Surgery has been well developed in allopathic system. At the same time medicines used in surgery has to be developed based on energy medicine systems. Anaesthesia is one of the strong medicines that cause side effects of nervous system. Ways to be found to reduce the chemical medicines and replacing with the energy medicines.

Researchers:

Dr. Albert P. Krueger said that this world of science may be forgiven for having failed for so long to take ions seriously as a major influence on life. This is a sad feeling for a person who did lot of research on the subject of negative ions and proved its use to the world and this is a low cost technology compared to the cost of modern medicine. Dr. Krueger predicted that we should someday regulate the ion level indoors much as we now regulate temperature and humidity. Ironically, today's air-conditioned buildings, trains and planes frequently become

supercharged with harmful positive ions because of the metal
blowers, filters and ducts of air-conditioning systems

Fred Soyka, a Canadian engineer and business executive, who
had spent around twelve years in Geneva, Switzerland, where
he faced his health problem due to the "Witches Winds" of the
city. He is sensitive to positive ions and hence the environment
created by the wind made his life, like those of many other
residents of the city of Geneva unbearable. In the hunt to find
the reason of his bad health, whenever he would set foot in
Geneva, he started his research and found a breakthrough that
directed him to a unique subject of Ions and how they affect
you, me and all around us. He wrote the book "Ion Effect"
in 1973 at the age of 42. He ends his book with a note that
"governments have to do something to relieve the distress of
people who get affected by positive ions. The real use of nature
only lies with the people like us".

Basics of a person to be developed:

When the seed of a plant is in a good soil it will start to grow
well. If proper manure is fed, and watered in time and kept
in a good environment, the plant will grow well. Develop the
plant and its internals to be healthy and do not care about
insects and pests. The innate strength of the plant will resist
the attack by insects. Same way strengthening the basic health
of the person will reduce the diseases. Add strength to the
fundamentals of human race by improving the base the soil,
environment, plants and animals. Then nature will take care
of all the opponents for good human health.

Only when we use the nature, we will know the nature and
we will know how the nature is helping us and that would
continue to help us. Add strength to the fundamentals of
human race by improving the base the soil, environment,

plants and animals. Then nature will take care of all the opponents for good human health.

Cosmic energy, the energy of the nature
is as necessary as water and air to
Humans, Animals, Plants and the Soil.

Cosmic energy will energize the earth forever.
We, the people of the earth, shall utilize
the energy for our benefits
if we want our
future generations to survive and be healthy.

References

1. **Life around**
- Becker, Robert O. – Body electric
- http://cosmicloti.com/tag/universal-energy/
- Dr. Charles Wallach – "Ion Controversy – A scientific Appraisal" -2010
- Fred Soyka – "The Ion effect – How air electricity rules your life and Health" – Bantam books
- Norman cousins "Anatomy of Illness" by Rane Dubos in preface.
- Tompkins, peter - "The Secret life of the plants" -Earthpulse press-2002
- Jean-Paul – Journal of Condensed Matter Nuclear science 7 -2012

2. **Around us**
- Bise winds of Geneva - http://www.weatheronline.co.uk/reports/wind/The-Bise.htm
- Bora - http://www.weatheronline.co.uk/reports/wind/The-Bora.htm
- Chinook and health - http://www.migraines.org/about_media/helthsct.htm
- Foehn - http://www.summitpost.org/foehn-effect/466432
- Haboob - http://www.weatheronline.co.uk/reports/wind/Haboob.htm
- Hayanon-What are cosmic rays
- Dr. Kruger A.P.-Report on negative ions-1967

- Mistral - http://www.frenchentree.com/holidays-in-france/weather/the- infamous -mistral-wind -in-provence/
- Sankaran- http://www.indiastudychannel.com/forum/128075-Karkitakam-adreaded-month-for-Kerala-people.aspx
- Srikumar – Kolar Gold field, unfolding the untold- 2014
- Thar desert - http://www.newworldencyclopedia.org/entry/Thar_Desert
- Wahlin, Lars – Atmospheric electrostatics, Colutron Research coprortion-1985

3. **Cosmic energy**
- Ken Wilbur- "The Spectrum of Consciousness"
- Siingh, Devendra and Singh RP-"The role of cosmic rays in the Earth's atmospheric processes" - Pramana-Journal of Physics – Jan 2010
- http://en.wikipedia.org/wiki/Cosmic_ray
- Negative Ion Report: The CBS Nightly News, Feb 14, 1995

4. **Posions Negions**
- Blenau, Wolfgang - Seratonin receptor technologies - Humana press Springer-2015
- Ermakov,V.I et al - Ion balance equation in the atmosphere –Journal of Geophysical Research – Vol 102 Oct. 1997
- Full moon effect - http://www.policeops.com/full-moon-ion-effect.htm
- Hayanon- 'What are cosmic rays' translated by Y.Noda et al.
- Ions - http://www.hyperstealth.com/ions.htm
- Ionisers - http://altered-states.net/index2.php?/ionizers/info.htm
- Seratonin - -http://www.causeof.org/sis.htm

- Robert M. Schoch, Robert Aquinas - Pyramid Quest: Secrets of the Great Pyramid and the Dawn of Civilization
- Siingh, Devendra and Singh RP-"The role of cosmic rays in the Earth's atmospheric processes" - Pramana-Journal of Physics – Jan 2010
- Soyka, Fred & Alan Edmonds (1991). "The Ion Effect" Bantam Books
- Walter,M –Early history of cosmic particle physics - European physics journal June-2012
- Winds effects - http://www.nytimes.com/1981/10/06/science/ions-created-by-winds-may-prompt-changes-in-emotional-states.html
- Zapping Airborne Salmonella and Dust - published in the March 2000 issue of Agricultural Research magazine.

5. Cosmic Energy in Health

- Bacteria eraser - http://www.djclarke.co.uk/ionisers-in-hospitals.html
- Barbara Brennan – "Hands of light, A guide to healing through the Human energy Field"
- Dr. Robert O. Becker Becker - The Body Electric: Electromagnetism And The Foundation Of Life - 1998
- Bhaskar - http://anatomictherapy.org/
- Borne- on migraine- http://stopthemigrainemadness.com/blog/migraine-and-the-weather/
- Boyle, John P. - NIC Generator Pattern Book. St. John press- 1975
- Robert O'Brien- Ions –Magic in the air - Rotarian –october-1960
- Case Adams - Asthma Solved Naturally: The Surprising Underlying Causes and Hundreds of natural strategies to beat asthma - Naturopath
- Carlos Castaneda – 'The Teachings Of Don Juan' -1968

- Daniels L. Satacy-"On the Ionization of Air for Removal of Noxious--IEEE Transactions on Plasma Science, Vol. 30, NO. 4, Aug. 2002
- Guy Cramer (1996) - Advanced Research on Atmospheric Ions and Respiratory Problems -by Sept. 2,1996
- Herd D.J. - Book- 'Zen & the Art of Pond Building'
- Holt, Peter S., Mitchell, Baily et al – Use of Negative air ionization for reducing airborne levels of Salmonella Enterica serovar enteritidis in a room containing infected caged layers- Applied poultry sciences- 1999
- Jones, D.P - Effect of long-term ionized air treatment on patients with bronchial asthma – Thorax -1976
- Krueger AP, Reed EJ - Biological impact of small air ions.-- Science. 1976 Sep 24;193(4259):1209-13. www.envirohealthtech.com/researchions.htm
- Mitchell, B.W - Reducing Airborne Pathogens, Dust and Salmonella Transmission in Experimental Hatching Cabinets Using an Electrostatic Space Charge System-poultry science-2002
- NASA use - http://www.mysticmarvels.com/benefits2.html
- Newton, Robert –Book- 'Pathways to God : Experiencing the Energies of the Living God in Your Everyday Life'
- Perez et al. (2013) : Air ions and mood outcomes: a review and meta-analysis. BMC Psychiatry 2013 13:29.
- Rachel Yarmolinsky A BRIGHTER OUTLOOK FOR SAD PATIENTS –Nov 2008- http://asp.cumc.columbia.edu/psych/articles/Article_Display.asp?ID=70
- Rosalind Tan - The Truth About Air Electricity & Health: A guide on the use of air ionization and other natural approaches-2013

- Shargawi. Sensitivity of Candida albicans to negative air ion streams - Journal of Applied Microbiology Journal of Applied Microbiology, Volume 87, Issue 6, on line on 25 DEC 2001
- Silverman, Daniel and Igo H. Kornbleuh. - Effect of artificial Ionization and the EEG- A Preliminary Report - Silverman EEG Clin. Neurophysiol., 1957
- Soyka, Fred & Alan Edmonds (1991). "The Ion Effect" Bantam Books
- Terman, Michael Ph.D., and Jiuan Su Terman, Ph.D. (1995) - Journal of Alternative and Complementary Medicine, 1:87-92, 1995 http://www.nalusda.gov/ttic/tektran/data/000008/54/0000085456.html
- Wang Wei –A study of negative air ion concentration in various environments in summer - Anhui Institute of Architecture-2014- http://www.ahjzu.edu.cn/s/33/t/45/cf/c0/info53184.htm
- Watson - http://www.zoominfo.com/p/Bernard-Watson /36336713
- Watson (2008) - http://www.primaltherapy.com/how-we-changed-serotonin-levels-naturally.php

6. **Health and disease**
- LEAH ZERBE-on TEFLON-http://www.rodales organiclife.com /home/ nonstick-cookware-teflon-dangers - FEBRUARY 14, 2013
- Teflon - http://www.spiritofhealthkc.com/wp/wp-content/uploads/2014/03/TEFLON-Teflon-Can-Cause-Birth-Defects-and-Infertility.pdf - TEFOL causing infertility.
- Bisong Guo and Andrew Powell –a book- "Listen to your body - the wisdom of dao", 2002 Hawaii press.
- Jaggi vasudev - https://rememberwhoweare.wordpress.com/2011/09/23/sadhguruquotes/
- Schuessler - The Twelve Tissue Remedies of Schüssler (5th ed.) by William, Dewey Boericke publishing.

- Kennedy, Martin Alexander -Mendel-diseases— Encyclopedia -of-life sciences. 2001- Nature publishing group
- Bateson, William – Mendel's principles of Heredity - Cambridge University Press. 1902

7. **Food**
- Bjorklund, Ruth -The sense -Marshal Cavendish -2010
- Calories-meat-http://www.freedieting.com/tools/calories_in_meat.htm
- Diet - http://www.cnpp.usda.gov/Publications/DietaryGuidelines/2010/PolicyDoc/PolicyDoc
- Digestion disorders - http://www.webmd.com/digestive-disorders/bowel-transit-time
- Food calories - http://www.scientificamerican.com/article/how-do-food-manufacturers/
- Guyton AC, Hall JE - Textbook of medical physiology – 2006
- Hollick, Julian Crandall - http://www.npr.org/templates/story/story.php?storyId=17134270
- Marsh,steve - http://www.theguardian.com/environment/2015/mar/26/gm-crop-farmer-told-to-reveal-if-he-was-backed-by-monsanto-in-legal-battle
- Rizaa, Robert team, Encyclopedia of food – A guide to healthy nutrition, Academic press, 2002
- WDDTY Asthma manual

8. **Medicines**
- Life extension – http://www.forbes.com/sites/john lechleiter/2012/05/22/extend-life-expectancy-and-reduce-deaths-yes-we-can/
- Marmor, Theodore.R – The politics of Mdicine.2nd ed. 2000- Aldine de gruyter press Newyork
- Rob Knight -Scientific American -March.2025
- Summer, Carl – A weakness in bactera' s fortress. - Scientific American 2015- Jan

- Wiki-history of medicine - https://en.wikipedia.org/wiki/History_of_medicine

9. **Herbs, Plants and Minerals**
- Minerals, sources – http://www.emedicinehealth.com/minerals_their_functions_and_sources-health/article_em.htm
- Chandra, Suman – Biotechnology for medical plants –Springer - 2013
- Schuessler - The Twelve Tissue Remedies of Schüssler (5th ed.) by William, Dewey Boericke publishing. 1914

10. **Chemicals**
- Coupon Sherpa - http://phys.org/news/2010-01-chemical-additives-food.html
- Gitanjali Singh - Estimated Global, Regional, and National Disease Burdens Related to Sugar-Sweetened Beverage Consumption in 2010 – Circulation magazine of American Heart Association.
- Penicillin - http://www.drugs.com/penicillin.html
- Penicillin history - http://inventors.about.com/od/pstartinventions/a/Penicillin.htm
- Penicillin ban- http://www.sciencedaily.com/releases/2012/04/120405131431.htm
- Science daily - <www.sciencedaily.com/releases/2015/06 /150629162646.htm>.
- may also raise your diabetes risk, says Grogan. (Suzanne Fantar)
- Suzanne Fantar, Demand Media, http://healthyeating.sfgate.com/sodium-nitrate-vs-sodium-nitrite-9064.html
- Michael S. Reid, A Brief History of 1-Methyl cyclopropene, Horticultural science Feb-2008.
- Mercola -- MSG: Is This Silent Killer Lurking in Your Kitchen Cabinets. http://articles.mercola.com/sites/articles/archive/2009/04/21/

msg-is-this-silent-killer-lurking-in-your-kitchen-cabinets.aspx
- Courtney Hutchison- Not So (O)Lean: Eating Faux Fat Makes Rats Real Fat. http://abcnews.go.com/Health/Diet/eating-fake-fat-makes-real-fat-olestra-study/story?id=13893613

11. Energy in medicine
- Pon Sivar-2013 narration by a farmer, rice grower.
- Sankaran, Rajan – 'The other song'
- Azeemi, Khwaja Shamsuddin – Colour therapy Al kitab publications-2007

12. Energized medicine
- Dr. David Frawley, Dr. Subash Ranade, and Dr. Avinash Lele -- Ayurveda and marma therapy http://www.morihata.com/products/binchotan/
- Jing-Nuan Wu - An illustrated Chinese materia medica - Oxford University Press, Inc.- 2005
- DR. LOCKIE, ANDREW - Encyclopedia of Homeopthy -DH publishing- 2005
- Owen, David - Principles and Practice of Homeopathy Churchill Livingstone- Elsevier -2007
- Kandaswamy, Pillai N. 1979. History of Siddha Medicine. Madras.
- Narayanaswami, V. 1975. Introduction to the Siddha System of Medicine. Madras.
- NIS- Chennai http://nischennai.org/siddhamedicine.html
- Schuessler - The Twelve Tissue Remedies of Schüssler (5th ed.) by William, Dewey Boericke publishing. 1914
- TCM-Five element theory -http://www.calvindale.com/fivelements.html
- Zhanwen Liu - Essentials of Chinese Medicine -3 volumes- Springer-2009
- Unani-wiki - https://en.wikipedia.org/wiki/Unani

13. **Energy Activation**
- Beijing College-Essentials_of_chinese-Acupuncture - Foreign language press Beijing - 1980
- Claudia Focks –Atlas of acupuncture – Churchill Livingstone - 2008
- Douglas colligan - State energies hidden powers
- Gala, Dhiren- Be your own doctor with acupressure – Navneet publications India Ltd.- 2003
- Giovanni Macioci -The Practice of Chinese Medicines-Churchill Livingstone - 1994
- Longe, Jacqueline L. - Gale Encyclopedia of medicine –Gale group - 2002
- Lungs efficiency - http://www.normalbreathing.com/patterns-oxygen-extraction.php
- Qi –energy http://www.med-etacupuncture.org/english/articles/arch/arch.html
- Silva method - http://youmeworks.com/the-silva-method.html

14. **Energy as Medicine**
- Choa Kok Sui - Pranic Healing - Samuel Weiser -1990 http://negativeionshealth.com/index.php?option=com_content&view=article&id=112:the-role-of-ions-in-body-chemistry &catid =16& Itemid =127
- Healthy-water-life - http://www.healthywaterlife.com/cgi-bin/d.cgi/signup/eco_friendly_uses_kitchen.html
- Helps health - http://www.djclarke.co.uk/file04b.html
- How ioniser works - http://www.djclarke.co.uk/file08.html
- Negative ions - https://www.quantumbalancing.com/negative_ions.htm
- Pyramid power - http://www.pyramid-cafe.in/Power.html

- Pyramids   -   http://www.iempowerself. com/84_pyramid_power.html
- Pranic healing - https://pranichealing.com/what-pranic -healing

15. **Old and New**
- Blenau, Wolfgang and Baumann, Arnd – "Serotonin receptor technologies" www.cosmicawareness.org Duke, James A. - Dukes's handbook of Medicinal Plants of the Bible –CRC press -2008
- Ion generators in - http://www.djclarke.co.uk/file06. html
- Natasha - http://www.newscientist.com/article/dn 3228 -air- ionizers -wipe-out-hospital-infections.htm
- Natasha McDowell – "Air ionisers wipe out hospital infections" –New scientist -3 January 2003 by
- Negion generators - http://www.negativeiongenerators. com/negativeions.html
- Welton, Janus Aia Bbei - "The Living Elements of Healthy Building Design"

16. **Future**
- "American Health demographics and spending of Health care consumers" –New Strategist publications-2010
- Bos JD1, Meinardi MM – "The 500 Dalton rule for the skin penetration of chemical compounds and drugs" – Experimental Dermatology -June 2000
- Chopra, Deepak – "Perfect health" -1990
- Ullman, Dana – "The Homeopathic Revolution: Why Famous People and Cultural Heroes Choose Homeopathy" - North Atlantic Books - 2007
- UMM - http://umm.edu/health/medical/altmed/ treatment/herbal-medicine